G000160351

The Right Way to Eat

The Right Way to Eat

to feel good – or even better

MIRIAM POLUNIN

J. M. Dent & Sons Ltd
London Melbourne Toronto

First published 1978

Printed in Great Britain by
Biddles Ltd, Guildford, Surrey
and bound at the
Aldine Press, Letchworth, Herts
for
J. M. Dent & Sons Ltd
Aldine House, Albemarle Street, London

This book is set in 11 on 11 pt VIP Baskerville

British Library Cataloguing in Publication Data
Polunin, Miriam
The right way to eat.
1. Diet
I. Title
613.2 RA784

ISBN 0-460-04319-6

Contents

Acknowledgments

I'd like to thank Ivan, my husband, who has helped me so much, and *Here's Health* magazine, which has generously allowed me to use material taken from my articles for *Here's Health*.

1. How Do You Feel Today?

Nowadays, we all feel we have a right to live a long time, and to be healthy for most of it. These expectations are based on a rosy national self-image of well-dressed cheerful families, bright clean homes and modern medicines that can tackle almost anything – a television-advertisement atmosphere of security and efficiency.

But the truth is different. Lots of young people get ill, and lots of people die before reaching retirement age or very soon afterwards. And even more of us spend most of our days feeling far from our best – not dramatically ill, but off-colour. Look around you at your family, friends and work colleagues and you'll see the proof that we are not the hale and hearty people we'd like to think we are. Look at any doctor's waiting-room, or the waiting-list for hospital specialist appointments. Look at the cost of the National Health Service, as the demands upon it increase instead of, as first expected, diminishing with prosperity. **Most ill health isn't a question of luck. A very big proportion of illnesses and early deaths is caused by the way we live, not by heredity or by chance.**

These illnesses could be avoided by changing our living habits, especially as every year we know more clearly what habits affect which aspects of ill health. Many diseases nowadays are diseases of choice: we prefer to have them than to change our ways. The outstanding example is smoking, which everyone recognizes has to be paid for in ill health.

But although we are indignant about ill health in the 'prime of life', there is a vast amount of ill health amongst older people which we accept with unreasonable complacency. We think it is normal for people to lose their mobility and energy in old age, to suffer from arthritis, rheumatism and 'chestiness', to become overweight and to lose some of their mental alertness. It *isn't* normal. Most of these disabilities are not inevitable. They are frequently the results of many years of unhealthy living habits.

This book is about one of the most important ways in which people decide what their own health and length of life will be: what they eat. Every day, three times a day for most of us, we choose food which, little by little, adds up to what we will become and how we will feel. In the past, most people's meals were dictated to them by their pocket. That narrow choice was even narrower before the Victorian era. Until then, people's menus were further restricted by the food which was locally and seasonally available, with little of the vast transportation, processing and preservation of food which give us so much variety today. Our generation is the first to have knowledge available about the effect of food on health, yet people are still unaware that deciding what to eat is also deciding on their health. We eat certain things because we like them, but these likings have usually been shaped by social habit and family background.

Social conditioning is very rigid: people can feel quite sick at the thought of eating something like steak and kidney pie for breakfast, even if they would welcome it three hours later. And they think someone very strange for making unusual combinations: for instance turkey and cranberry sauce is normal, but sausages and strawberry jam is breaking a social pattern. Class plays a part too: some foods are more highly valued than others, not because they taste nicer or are more nutritious, but because they cost more or carry an association of nobility: there's no practical reason, for instance, why bony, skinny quails should be thought 'better' than chicken, but they are. People often react strongly, too, to a food they ate a lot of in childhood – they may hate it for the whole of their adult lives, or return to it compulsively, finding it carries with it pleasant emotions or even a feeling of security.

Examples like these add up to an obvious yet often ignored fact. When people choose food, they choose more than calories and taste. As food advertisers realize, shoppers are after emotional as much as physical satisfaction, conjuring up memories, confirming a social image for themselves, carrying on traditions.

These are strong influences. But I don't believe it is a waste of time trying to make people aware of the other choice involved – the choice of their future health. Eating food you like, for whatever reason, and eating healthily are not incompatible. And the claim that ordinary people's eating habits are hopelessly fixed and immovable is not only patronizing, but demonstrably wrong. For people's tastes in food have changed enormously in the past century alone, and are changing now. And although it seems that recent changes have been for the worse from a nutritional point of view, there's no reason why future changes should not be for the better. After all, since the first vitamin was isolated only sixty years ago it is only recently that we've known what 'the better' means in food and health terms.

This book sets out to answer the question: how should I eat to stay healthy, get healthier and – just as important – feel good? I want to show how our everyday decisions about meals are worth looking at and perhaps changing. These decisions may seem too small to matter at the time, but, in total, they can repay you with years of feeling good, looking good and – not a sensationalist but a sensible claim – extra life.

I'm not saying that people *ought* to change their eating habits, and certainly not that they should be made to. What I am saying is that people should be aware of the big part food plays in health. Once they know what they are choosing, it is up to them to decide whether to make changes, or to go on as they are. In my view, they *can't* make up their own minds until they know the position. The choice is not between healthy food that tastes horrid and delicious but unhealthy food. The changes that can make or break health are often small, undramatic and quite easy to fit into existing likes and dislikes. The fact that we have so much choice leaves us more room to go wrong – and much more opportunity to go right. We could – we can – be super-nourished, super-healthy, super-looking. Just think of a day when you felt at your very best . . . wouldn't it be good to feel and look your best every day?

SO WHERE ARE WE GOING WRONG?

The magazine I edit decided to carry out a survey of why people are interested in health. One of the likely reasons was that they were dissatisfied with their own physical well-being So when we worked out a questionnaire to be put to thousands of people chosen at random in the street, we thought we would ask them how healthy they felt. But how do you measure that? We didn't want to know what their blood pressure, health record or cholesterol levels were – but how good they felt.

The answer to the problem came from one of our contributors, naturopath Joan Lay. At one of her lectures, she asked the audience (who weren't patients) how they would rate their healthiness out of a maximum of 100 per cent. Most of the people there – people who were not ill, or medically-minded or trained – found no difficulty in giving themselves a rating – between 60 and 80 per cent. I was fascinated at this awareness by people of how good they felt. Of course, it might not be a reflection of their physical condition or life expectancy, but it was a true picture of their well-being (or otherwise). Clearly 'otherwise' played an important part. This percentage may not be terribly impressive. And yet I think that day-to-day well-being is terribly important. In my view it's even more important than living a long time. It's feeling good that makes life worth living.

After listening carefully to people I meet, and reading the hundreds of questions sent in every month to the magazine, I have come to the conclusion that very few people feel good most of the time. Most people seem to spend at least half their time feeling well below perfect: not ill, but not well. The commonest ailments I meet are feeling lacking in energy, 'throat-y', 'headache-y', bloated, acidic or otherwise uncomfortable round the tummy, feeling they are just coming down with/recovering from some 'bug', stiff, 'backache-y', or just unduly and persistently tired. On top of this vague 'unwellness' there are the more concrete diseases of which these symptoms are a weaker reflection. We have a longer life expectancy than our great grandparents – but does that mean we are healthier? We live longer not because we live more healthily but because we have improved techniques of childbirth and infant care, and because we have largely eliminated the epidemic diseases which used to kill large numbers of people. Those diseases were caused and spread by ignorance of the importance of hygiene, particularly water hygiene. The elimination of these mass killers is a marvellous achievement. But our basic state of health is nothing to be proud of, considering the improved food supplies and health knowledge available to us. Here are some of the diseases which are so common that most people almost regard them as normal:

allergies and hay fever
appendicitis†
catarrh and sinus
'chestiness' – from asthma
to bronchitis
colds, coughs and 'flu'
constipation
cystitis and other urinary

infections†
dental decay
gallstones†
haemorrhoids
hernias
indigestion and flatulence
intestinal disorders, particularly diverticulosis and mucous colitis (irritable colon)†
menstrual disorders
migraine†
poor eyesight
prostate problems
repeated headaches
rheumatism and arthritis
skin disorders, from acne to psoriasis
stomach and duodenal ulcers†
thrush and other vaginal infections†
varicose veins

Taken more seriously, because they handicap or threaten life, yet still taken remarkably for granted, are angina,† diabetes,† high blood pressure,† pneumonia, severe overweight†. The killers, like heart disease,† cancer, thrombosis, are enormously and rightly feared, but are still seen as a natural part of life which just has to be lived – or more properly, died – with. Well, they *are* a part of British life today – because this whole depressing list is so common. But this amazing assumption – that human beings just do get these illnesses – is a dreadful and pathetic illusion. It is dreadful, because it is a kind of brainwashing, which stops people making any attempt to avoid all this pain and life-ruining illness. It is pathetic because the evidence that these diseases are *not* inevitable is so obvious.

Whole populations in other countries simply don't get certain Western ailments. They get other illnesses, but they do prove that ours are not man's universal heritage. Thailand, for instance, proves that tooth decay isn't inevitable: half the population doesn't have to lose all its own teeth as they do in Britain. African and Asian countries prove that appendicitis, diverticulosis, constipation and varicose veins belong to a life style, not to life itself. Nor is it a question of race. Japanese Americans and Black Americans, for instance, suffer from all the 'Western diseases', although their racial brothers in Japan and Africa don't. And our own history proves that it isn't climate or landscape that makes the difference: many of the diseases on my depressing list were rare here only a century ago. Yes, they were known – it's not

† = diseases we know are increasing in frequency.

a question of wrong diagnosis. But they were very, very rare.

Take appendicitis, for instance: what better example of a disease most of us imagine to be entirely a question of luck? The proof that it isn't has been best presented by A. Elliot-Smith, former Senior Surgeon at Radcliffe Infirmary, Oxford. He was personally convinced of the 'newness' of certain diseases which seemed to have appeared only near the beginning of this century. But, as he wrote in *Just Consequences**, 'When a new disease is announced it is often suggested that this is an old disease newly recognized, and that the bedside clinician of a hundred years ago was often unable correctly to diagnose the malady. There may be some truth in this contention, but at least the pathologist carrying out the examination after death was usually able to say what had been the cause of death.' So Mr Elliot-Smith decided to use the fact that he worked at a hospital which had kept records since its foundation in 1770 to see how the new diseases had arrived.

Appendicitis was known in the nineteenth century, because it was described in medical literature. But in the 125 years between its opening and 1895, the Radcliffe hospital dealt with only between five and ten cases of appendicitis a year. By 1905, there were 40 cases a year; by 1930, 300 a year, and by 1970, over 500 cases a year. Ulcers were his second point of focus: Radcliffe records only mentioned them in 1891. And because ulcers have always been a reason for discharge from the army, there were good records of ulcers from there too. In the seventeen months from August 1914 to the end of 1915, there were 709 discharges on the grounds of ulcers. In the twenty-eight months from September 1939 to the end of 1941 (in a similar size army), instead of about 1400 discharges as one might have expected, there were 23,500 men discharged because they were found to have ulcers. You can't blame it on the army food either! First, army food was better in the Second World War, and secondly, most of the men were found to have had the ulcers *before* entering the army. Similar increases can also be shown for all the diseases I have marked on my list with an ominous cross!

What about the most ominous word of them all, cancer? I haven't marked it with a cross, because some cancers have

* *Just Consequences* is an excellent collection of essays on food and health by distinguished medical and food researchers, published by Charles Knight & Co., 1971.

become more common, and others, less common. On the increase in epidemic fashion is cancer of the lung, and rising gradually are, for instance, cancer of the bowel and breast. Examples of types of cancer decreasing slightly are cancer of the stomach and intestine.

You can't dodge the facts of these increases by pointing to increased population – the rises far exceed our extra citizens. And you can't use that other old chestnut, that people didn't live long enough to get such illnesses. Most of my list of everyday nasties are just as common among young and 'prime of life' people as they are among the elderly. Besides, the life expectancy of *adults* hasn't risen so much: in 1841, a man of fifty could expect to reach seventy. In 1967, he could expect to live to seventy-three.

Below is another table* to finish off the depressing facts I feel compelled to rub in (otherwise how am I to break the strong belief that's instilled into us that we are really much healthier than our forefathers?) It shows what our chances – yours and mine – are of developing some of the commonest of these 'new' diseases – plus some not-so-new to Britain, but less common in many other countries.

If you're a man:

1 in 4 will develop chronic bronchitis
1 in 4 will get cancer, of which
  1 in 30 will get cancer of the lung, and
  1 in 35 will get cancer of the stomach
1 in 5 will develop coronary heart disease
1 in 12 will be admitted to general hospital in a year
1 in 12 will have a peptic ulcer

If you're a woman:

1 in 4 will be regularly visiting their GP with a health
  problem that won't go away
1 in 5 will develop cancer, of which
  1 in 20 will have cancer of the breast
1 in 8 will have diabetes
1 in 14 will be admitted to general hospital in a year

But I don't think it should be necessary to quote statistics to prove to most of us that our health isn't as good as it should

* *Health Hazards in Middle Age – Statistics of the Risks*, Royal Society of Health Journal, April 1967. R. F. Logan.

be: we know if it isn't. And a lot of it has to do with food.

Do I have to convince you that food and health are almost the same thing? It should be obvious. We are all made up of millions of cells, and every moment, hundreds of chemical interactions are going on inside us to keep us ticking over. These cells are constantly dying, and new ones being formed to replace them. Most people seem to think that this process stops when we become fully grown, but it doesn't. The rate of turnover of cells slows down, but never stops. Food is the only source of all the raw materials that the body needs for this continual rebuilding, and for all the complicated functions that enable us to think, move, feel, see, hear, digest, sleep, react.

We already know at least forty substances which we must obtain from food to fuel these activities. That is to say, if even one is missing, we become seriously and perhaps fatally ill. The necessities we know of are grouped under carbohydrates, fats, proteins, minerals, vitamins and probably enzymes. Some are needed in large quantities, some we require only in very tiny amounts – a thousandth of a milligram, which in itself is only a thousandth part of a gram, which is roughly one thirtieth of an ounce, per day. Because most of us are hooked on the notion that bigger things are more important, we easily ignore the 'little 'uns' of nutrition. Yet the ill-effects when one of these is missing are just as devastating as if we're short of a 'major' food ingredient. Vitamin B12 is one such 'tiny' nutrient, but the anaemia which the lack of it will cause can kill just as surely as a lack of calcium, which we need hundreds of times more of per day.

All these forty food elements not only have to be available, but in the right proportions and combinations for the body to produce the right effects from them. Just like a cake mixture, you need lots of some ingredients, and hardly any of others, but too little or too much of just one item may ruin the whole recipe. **If we get the recipe right, the body will run as well as it can.** We will feel our best, act with maximum ease and efficiency. What better recipe for health and happiness? And as well as direct results of the lack of some essential food element there may be other, indirect, ill-effects. For once the body is not receiving the right 'fuel', it is more vulnerable to all kinds of illness.

We don't all need to be biochemists in order to choose food which contains the right food elements. Luckily, man is surrounded by foods which contain a selection of all the ingredients of the 'fuel' he needs. I use the word 'luckily' because even if we *were* all trained as biochemists, we wouldn't be able to pick out the foods to provide the ideal recipe for our bodies: we don't exactly know what the recipe is. Modern science has given us a lot of information about food values, so we know roughly what we should be looking for. On the other hand, anyone who claimed that he knew *exactly* how many grams of protein we need a day would be a liar – nobody does. But we have learned enough to know how complicated the body's needs are and to draw ourselves guidelines as to what food combination is likely to suit health best.

But if man has survived for so long without any of this knowledge, and if we are surrounded by foods which supply the kind of fuel we need, why do we need to bother about nutrition at all? Reason one: things go wrong. In fact, most of our knowledge about the importance of certain food elements is based on observation of what has happened when things have gone wrong. Think of how many tens of thousands of seamen died of scurvy before it was realized that it was related to food. Without the introduction of long voyages which were perfect laboratory testing grounds for finding what caused this fatal illness (which also happened, although less predictably, on dry land) how long would it have taken to recognize the importance of something special and essential in fruit and vegetables – the element later isolated and called ascorbic acid or vitamin C? The importance of iodine was realized because goitres were common in the people of the Black Forest area as a result of iodine deficiency in the soil and food grown in it. The observed effects of deficiency are thus the basis for all official figures of food needs.

But, you may say, things went wrong in the past because there wasn't enough food to go round, or it was badly distributed, but nowadays we all have plenty. Which leads to reason two: we have more food, but it is different food from that of the past. Again, I am not harking back to the good old days. For most people, they weren't. But the food of 200 years ago did contain all the food elements it possessed by nature when harvested. Ours doesn't. **We have learned how to change food to suit our convenience, and we have changed it and our eating habits almost beyond recognition.**

The food revolution: 1800

1800	Main foods for most people were bread, cheese, beer, meat, fish, root vegetables and cabbage family. Expensive but growing in popularity were tea, sugar and coffee which were all imported and subject to heavy taxes which made them luxury foods. There was only homegrown fruit, vegetables and meat. Flour was the main commodity; it was sieved wholemeal, so it retained all nutrients except some bran. No preserving methods except drying, salting or cheesemaking for milk.	Sugar consumption about 6lbs per year. Bread and flour about 370lbs per year, or about 1lb per day. Fat intake under 1oz per day. Low intake of fruit and vegetables, but what was eaten was locally grown and usually fresh. More bulk of food eaten but only slightly more calories, in spite of much higher calorie use for most people.
1810	Bottling as a method of food preservation was invented by Nicholas Appert a Parisian confectioner who won the prize Napoleon had offered in 1795 for the person who devised a successful food preserving method.	If calorie intake was high enough, diet provided enough nutrients except for iodine-deficient areas and sometimes vitamin D shortage, producing rickets.
1812	Tinned cannisters were used instead of bottles by a London firm, Donkin, Hall and Gamble. Very expensive as each tin was hand made: mainly used for naval expeditions.	
	Grocers multiplied to supply growing urban communities. They sold a very limited range, almost all basic foods: tea, coffee, chocolate, spices, sugar, rice, sago, semolina, dried fruit, nuts and a few more. There were virtually no branded, ready-made foods in shops.	
1831	First commercial biscuit factory was started by Jonathan Dodgson Carr, son of a Kendal grocer.	
1830s	Potatoes joined staple foods. Railways started up on a countrywide scale, but were not used extensively for food transport because the travel cost made the food uncompetitive with local supplies.	Arrival of railways first step in move to centralized food production, rather than local. New need was for food that could travel without spoiling.
1841	First commercial jam factory was set up in Soho by Messrs. Crosse and Blackwell. Before this jam was made at home or bought from local shops. Commercial manufacture only became practical because of lower sugar prices as taxes were cut in '36 and '44.	Sugar consumption jumped to about 17lbs per person per year in 1844; rose to 34lbs by 1854, 42lbs by 1864 with removal of tax.
1845	More reductions in sugar tax followed over next 10 years. Railway transport continued to develop.	More fruit and vegetables eaten, but otherwise trend moved towards processed foods with losses of vitamins and minerals. Branded foods began to appear in shops. Tea consumption soared from 1833 level of 1¼lbs per head a year to 3¼lbs by 1863. Potatoes important: about 300lbs per person a year.
1864	Tax on sugar and tea removed, resulting in big jump in consumption of both, and of sugar-based foods such as jam, chocolate and sweets.	
1866	Solid chocolate first sold, made by John Cadbury and his brother.	
1869	Margarine first experimentally made by Mege-Mouries in France.	
1870s	Tinned meat technique developed to bring meat from Australia cheaply. It cost the equivalent of about 2½p per lb bones, about a third of UK meat price.	

	Roller mills introduced for grinding wheat. They quickly replaced most stonegrinding mills because they were faster and made whiter flour, really white instead of sieved wholemeal.	
1880	Refrigerated shipping developed for meat, butter, lard and bacon imports, so these foods became much cheaper as supply improved. Tinned food became generally available. More preservative chemicals used.	Cheaper fat and protein encouraged switch from potatoes, bread and flour. Bread intake down to 280lbs a year. New roller-milled flour was without wheat germ oil, bran and many vitamins and minerals. Cut in fibre intake from bran because of milling method, and because of falling bread intake. Fat intake still restricted by poverty, meat about 4oz per day. Sugar intake up to 85lbs per person per year. Tea consumption still rising. Switch to processed foods, encouraged by better transport.
1890	Refined breakfast cereals (Cornflakes) invented by Dr Kellogg at Battle Creek sanitarium, Michigan.	
1900	Sugar prices continued to be low, so that sugar and fat became cheap foods after centuries of being costly.	
1920	Spray drying and roller drying developed to produce 'instant' powdered foods such as milk and coffee. Vacuum drying applied to vegetables. Lorries arrived in force.	
1930	Frozen food became commercially successful. For the first time, the seasons became much less important in food supply.	
1940s	First period when almost every westerner had not only enough to eat, but a choice of food. Food processing industry developed fast as trend began to produce foods in large-scale plants, from where it was distributed countrywide. This brought the need for food to be durable under storage and transport: the need for food to keep longer than it would naturally encouraged the growth of the additive industry.	Sharp drops in potato, bread and flour intakes, replaced by sugar, fat, as incomes rose. Bread and flour down to about 150lbs per person a year (up during war years to 240–50lbs), sugar topped 110lbs (under rationing, 70–80lbs), fat over 50lbs (30–40lbs during rationing). Potatoes down to 190lbs (up to 280 during war).
1950s on	Convenience foods became more and more important, following the sharp decline in domestic service, equally sharp rise in number of working women. Additive industry produced hundreds of new compounds and new uses to make food keep longer, look more uniform or attractive.	Bread and flour intake down to about 110lbs per year, still dropping. Potatoes down to under 200lbs. Sugar: about 126lbs (about 5½oz per day). Fat: about 114lbs (5oz per day). Meat up to 135lbs (about 6 oz a day) – and protein from eggs has trebled.

NET RESULTS

1. Sugar up 20 times.
2. Fat up at least 5 times.
3. Protein up slightly.
4. Fibre or roughage down by about half: cereal fibre reduced to negligible amount, but fibre from vegetable and fruit up.
5. Almost all food is processed, with changes in its basic properties.
6. To help centralized production, use of additives has soared.

While change isn't wrong just because it *is* change, if we move away from the balance that exists in nature, and we don't know exactly what we are moving to, we must consider carefully what our chances are of improving on nature. We may have learned a lot about the links between food and health, but we've learned even more how much we don't know yet. We've learned how to dissect food and identify many elements of it – but we haven't learned how to put it together. The table (above) shows some of the important changes in food and eating patterns which have taken place in the past 150 years. Of course, some have been improvements. But some are known to be closely related to our 'new' health problems. And others are suspected of being related to them. The changes are many, but in my view when we're looking at food and health, they boil down to two major trends – the concentration of calories in our food, and the amount we process it – which I intend to discuss in the following two chapters.

2. More Calories, Less Bulk

The twentieth-century table has been summed up by Dr James Lambert Mount in a neat sentence: "Food is richer, softer and sweeter than ever before." The net result of all the changes in incomes, social conditions, food production and transport is that we have drastically changed the way we get our energy.

There are four elements in food which provide the human body with calories – our way of measuring the energy our body can derive from food. The four elements are carbohydrates, fats, proteins and alcohol. The mainstay of the British, and most other, populations until this century was carbohydrates. Carbohydrate is almost a dirty word today. People automatically think of carbohydrates as 'fattening', and imagine plates of cakes, pudding and sticky buns. Despite their common image, however, carbohydrates are not 'just stodge'. They provide calories, but no more than other food elements. Carbohydrates (which include all the starch and sugar substances) provide the same number of calories per ounce as proteins. That is about 4 calories per gram, or 112 per ounce (= about 28 grams). That's much less than alcohol (7 calories per gram) and less than half as much as fats (9 calories per gram, or 252 per ounce). These figures are for the food elements by themselves, but of course in natural foods, they are usually all mixed up. Most natural foods contain some carbohydrate, fat and protein, together with a large percentage of water and, in natural carbohydrate foods, fibre.

But our lowest calorie foods, such as lettuce, cucumber, carrots and fruit, are much closer than the sticky buns to being exclusively carbohydrate. In fruit and vegetables, and in grain foods like wholemeal bread, brown rice or porridge, the carbohydrates are generously diluted with water and fibre. Most greengroceries are between 80 and 95 per cent water, while wholemeal bread, rice or spaghetti contain up to 40 per cent water. These foods (provided they are whole grain cereals, and unprocessed vegetables) also contain fibre – structural material which doesn't provide calories, but does make food bulkier. The result is that we have to eat a large amount of this kind of food to get a lot of calories.

But in puddings and pies, for example, an ultra-concentrated, water-less and fibre-less carbohydrate is used – sugar. It takes about six pounds of sugar beet (where the sugar is diluted with water and fibre just as in any other vegetable) to produce a pound of sugar crystals. But you can eat an ounce of sugar – the same calories as in six times more sugar beet or other vegetables – almost without noticing. The volume has been taken away from the calories.

It is the *concentrated* sugar in cakes and puddings which pushes up the calories you get per ounce – not the fact that they contain carbohydrate. Don't forget, too, that puddings, etc. are usually rich in ultra-calorific fats – the only food with more calories than sugar – and baked items like cakes, biscuits, pastry and pies contain quite a lot of protein too. These other elements add just as many calories as carbohydrate.

It's important to realize how brainwashed we've been with the idea that protein is somehow a 'good' thing, and carbohydrates 'bad'. In calorie terms, it is 'concentrated' – food with little bulk per calorie – which should be the dirty word, especially for those with weight problems. It's so easy to eat too much of the concentrated foods like sugar and fat, because their physical bulk doesn't make one feel full.

Weight problems were something people in 1800 had few of – even though about 80 per cent of their calorie intake came from carbohydrate. Their carbohydrates were almost all of the diluted kind – with bread, porridge and root vegetables dominating most people's meals. (If you really think carbohydrates are fattening, look at Chinese or Japanese people, who have plenty to eat, most of it carbohydrate – but diluted carbohydrate in rice and vegetables. Their figures are far more svelte than those of high protein nations.) The remaining 20 per cent of their calorie intake was split roughly half and half between protein and fat.

This division of calories can be best seen in bread. White bread contains about 70 calories an ounce, wholemeal only about 63. An ounce of white bread contains these approximate* proportions of the three calorie-giving elements:

1 ounce white bread (= 28 grams)

Carbohydrates	(14½ grams)	:	58 calories	(82%)
Fats	(2/5 gram)	:	3½ calories	(5%)
Proteins	(2¼ grams)	:	9 calories	(13%)
Total		:	70½ calories	

Other grains show similar proportions, although unrefined grains and wholemeal bread contain slightly more fat and more protein. The other main foods of 1800 were cheese, meat, fish and milk – which provided fats and proteins with little carbohydrates – and vegetables – which provided little fat and less protein. The rough balance was maintained at carbohydrate 80 per cent: fat 10 per cent: protein 10 per cent.

Although this balance of food was not chosen, but the result of circumstances, everything we know about the body's needs suggests that it was a satisfactory balance, provided enough food was available. But many people didn't have enough food and were so near starvation that they ate virtually nothing but the cheapest source of calories, bread.

Given the right quantity of food to provide enough calories for energy, however, the balance included enough fats and proteins for their essential bodily functions. It was a balance based on the food the country grew – a balance which had remained stable for hundreds of years.

But it wasn't what everyone ate. Richer people had a different tradition. And they chose what they liked, not simply what they could afford. In their choice lies the origin of the term 'rich food'. What do you think of as rich food? Cream, sauces, lots of butter, foods like duck and pâté? Rich food really means food with more fat in it. More meat, more dairy foods, more eggs.

Richer people also ate more sugar, which was a really expensive luxury up to 130 years ago: in 1780, for instance, a pound of 'double-refined' sugar – nearest to our white sugar – cost 1s 3d (compared to the typical weekly wage of perhaps 15 shillings). And there was a third way in which the rich

* Bread made wholly from North American wheat has more protein; most bread in the UK is a mixture of North American and European wheat, approximately 50:50.

were the forerunners of modern tastes. They ate the whitest bread, made from the most finely sieved flour.

These were three trends which spread. In spite of the poverty of the majority of the population, the rich man's traditions came within reach of more and more of the population. By a combination of trade and technical developments, and by chance, the foods which had been costly and exclusive became among the cheapest.

Britain's domestic output of fats had always been low – it still is – but the opening up of a high volume international trade and cold storage brought a plentiful supply of fats from abroad. Sugar, too, instead of being exclusive luxury, became one of the cheapest sources of calories. And the development of a new method of refining flour made white bread, so long the status symbol of the rich, the norm for everyone.

Over a hundred years later, almost everyone chooses what they eat. The amount of fat eaten has risen relentlessly (except in wartime), and fats now provide about 42 per cent of the average person's calories. The rise of sugar in our affections has been even steeper: the present intake of about 5½ ounces per person per day is about twenty times as much as people ate in 1800. Sugar from food and drink now provides about 22 per cent of our daily calories.

Fats, at about 250 calories per ounce, are our most concentrated food. Sugar, at 112 calories per ounce, is our second most concentrated. Neither occur in a pure form in nature, but we've learned how to extract and therefore concentrate them. Almost two-thirds of our calories now come from these most concentrated foods.

While we're moving towards more concentrated foods, the third rich man's tradition, white bread, has taken even more bulk out of our diet. The introduction of flour refining, together with people's move away from flour products towards sugar, has substantially reduced the amount of food we swallow to get our calories. Taking bread alone, we know that a typical working man would have eaten at least 1 lb of wholemeal bread a day. It sounds a fantastic amount, but its 1000-odd calories are no more than you would get from a large fried steak and chips. That bread would in addition provide about 50 grams – nearly two ounces – of dietary fibre. Today, white bread contains so little fibre that the same amount eaten would give only 12½ grams of fibre. But we don't eat the same amount of any kind of bread: we eat sugary or creamier foods to get our calories instead. They, along with meat, eggs, cheese, milk and fish, contain no fibre at all.

What are the consequences of the move to concentrated, less bulky foods – and why do we choose them? Let us look at the effects of sugar and fats, and finally at the role of fibre in our diet.

SUGAR

Sugar is a word with two meanings. First it is our name for a particular family of chemical substances within the carbohydrate family. Secondly it is used to refer to just one member of this family, sucrose – the refined sugar we buy. This is the sugar we eat so much of – a combination of two other sugars, glucose and fructose. It is important to ask what is the difference between sugar in the amounts in which it occurs in naturally sweet foods – grapes, apples, sugar cane – and the way in which we eat it. The answer is that it is just the amount we eat. Does it matter if we eat a lot of sugar? Yes, because it changes our whole nutritional balance in the following ways:

★ because people eat a lot of sugar, they eat that much less of foods which can supply the forty-odd other elements essential to our health. With sugar supplying nearly a quarter of our calories, that means that our total food is only supplying three quarters of the vitamins, minerals, fibre and other elements it would normally.

★ because you can eat a lot of calories from sugar without feeling full, you can get fat on it easily.

★ because sugar is the cause of tooth decay, we have worse teeth than ever before.

★ because the digestion of sugar requires thiamin (vitamin B1), eating a lot of sugar pushes *up* our need for this vitamin, while at the same time, pushing *out* the foods which might supply it. Vitamin B1 is essential to the nervous system. It can't be stored by the body so even a few days of deficiency quickly produces symptoms, such as moodiness, irritation and constipation. By the way, most foods such as dates, which are naturally sugary also contain vitamin B1 – unless they have been refined.

★ because eating a lot of sugar produces abnormal body reactions, the result can be moodiness. Sugar in its concentrated, refined form is very quickly digested, and absorbed as glucose into the bloodstream. The level of sugar in our bloodstreams goes up whenever we eat, and a steady blood sugar level improves our concentration, abilities and mood. But concentrated sugar produces an abnormal 'high'. To turn sugar into energy, we need insulin from the pancreas. The sugar 'high' stimulates the pancreas, to produce a correspondingly high amount of insulin. This quickly clears the sugar from the bloodstream, resulting in a rapid fall in good mood and efficiency. This 'low' often hits people about two hours after a sugary meal – most often at 11 am, since breakfast is, as I shall mention later, a really sugary meal for most people.

These 'lows' produce a lack of energy which naturally encourages us to eat something sweet as a source of quick energy. This sets off a vicious circle. Eating a sugary diet can lead to switchback patterns in mood and efficiency. These can be extreme, with near euphoria, followed by dark moods and even blackouts.

For some people, the response to sugar is so sharp that their whole behaviour is dominated by it. But because sugar is such an everyday food, people may easily think it's all in the mind, and not realize the relationship. People have been known to be diagnosed as neurotic, and in one case, epileptic, whose symptoms disappeared within weeks of banning sugar from their meals.

⋆ because of its stimulant power, sugar can become an addiction. It's not too dramatic a word for the facts. People crave for sugar so much that they daren't open a box of chocolates, or a packet of sweet biscuits, 'because once I eat one, I can't stop until I've finished them'. Children will scream, throw tantrums and sulk over being refused sweets in a way they never would do over savoury foods. Many people prefer to buy sweets in small bars or quantities, because they recognize that they'll eat as much as they buy in a single session. No food dominates mood as sugar can.

⋆ in more and more of us, our pancreas eventually can't cope with the abnormally high, sudden demands for insulin. No meal based on natural foods makes such calls on it. When the pancreas stops providing the right amount of insulin, the result is diabetes.

⋆ sugar gives some people spots.

★ there are other charges of harmful effects made against sugar. The ones above are universally recognized, but others may be too, in time. At present, however, they are only interesting theories. Coronary heart disease is made more likely by a high sugar intake, according to some researchers. This is because a high sugar intake seems to encourage a high level of fats in the blood – a definite risk factor in heart disease.

Some surgeons specializing in intestinal disorders believe that a high level of sugar in food encourages the activity of harmful bacteria in the intestine. They believe that this explains the rising frequency of some intestinal diseases, and perhaps, cancer of the bowel.

A third health problem which may be connected to sugar is urinary and vaginal infections: sugar encourages an alkaline bias in the delicate acid/alkali balance of body secretions. The organisms which cause thrush, cystitis and other irritations thrive on this alkaline atmosphere. These infections are reaching epidemic proportions in some Western countries, aggravated by the adoption of nylon tights and underwear. Cutting sugar out of the diet sometimes helps recurrent cases, who don't benefit from drug treatment.

Action

Reducing the amount of sugar you eat automatically improves your health, because sugar is virtually the only 'empty calorie' food there is. Every time you replace some of it with another food, you are increasing your intake of the essential food elements – vitamins and minerals. Cutting down on sugar is a more effective slimming step than cutting down on bread, potatoes or other so-called fattening carbohydrates: a slice of bread, at 65 calories, is far more nutritious and satisfying than a 112-calorie ounce of sugar.

Here's a step-by-step plan for cutting down on sugar. Eating less sugar isn't a sort of monastic masochism. It need not cut you off from the rest of the world, or from your social life.

Step-by-step sugar-cutting plan

Step 1. Find out how much sugar you do eat by using the list of sugar in foods (p.24). Most people deny they eat a lot of sugar; and they don't eat a lot of sugar they add to food

Sugar in food

added sugar (sucrose) in common foods	
Food	*Sugar in ounces* (approximate)
2 sweet or chocolate biscuits	1/4
2oz chocolate bar	1
1 jam slice or doughnut	1/3
2oz slice of cake	2/3
1 1/4oz sugar-frosted cereal	1/4
1oz cornflakes, plain	1/10
6oz glass cola/soft drink	3/4
1 slice (3 1/2oz) fruit pie	3/4
4oz tinned fruit	1/3
1 helping (2 1/2oz) ice cream	1/2
1oz jam/marmalade	3/4
4oz jelly	3/4
4oz steamed pudding	1 1/3
4oz instant whip dessert	2/3
5oz milk pudding, e.g. rice	1/2
1 tsp sugar, rounded	1/4
1 yoghurt, fruit-flavoured (5oz)	2/3

themselves. But sugar lurks unseen in so many daily foods, that the 5½ ounce national daily average is quite easy to reach without realizing.

Don't try to cut down on sugar at all. Just add up your daily intake for a few days, using my list of the sugar in daily foods: you'll need to write down what you ate.

Step 2. From your list, you'll see where you get most of your daily sugar. You may find that you are getting most of your sugar from soft drinks – or tea – or from your evening dessert. It is different for different people. But looking at your list will show you where sugar can be reduced most effectively, and most conveniently for you.

Add up all the sugar you ate on the days you wrote it down, divide by the number of days, and you'll have your present sugar intake. Now use that to set a target, to halve that amount by this time next week.

Step 3. It's vital to accept that sugar is not essential to your quality of life. So doing without it is not a penance. It's helpful to remember all those generations of energetic, life-loving people who got on perfectly well without added refined sugar – although not without sweetness, since there are plenty of naturally sweet, but naturally diluted, foods such as fruit and honey. So when you start cutting down, don't let social pressures put you off. Just do it, don't feel you need to explain or justify your actions.

Step 4. One week later, check your sugar intake for another couple of days, to see if you have achieved your target. If you have, set yourself a new target: halve your current sugar intake again within the next week. This target will probably require more effort, and more careful planning. Here are some suggestions on how to avoid the sweeter things of life:

Breakfast is the sugariest meal of the day for most people. If you eat breakfast cereal, check the ingredients list to see if it contains sugar. The sweetest cereals are the sugar-coated types, followed by mueslis sold in supermarkets, followed by cornflakes and wheat biscuits. If possible, replace any sugared cereal with one with no sugar at all – such as Shredded Wheat, porridge, home-made muesli excluding sugar, or wheat germ. Second best is a bran cereal, since these are lower in sugar than most others.

Sugar on cereal is one of the major sources of sugar especially for children. If you can wean yourself off it gradually, that's best. Otherwise, try adding pre-cooked prunes, dried apricots, dates or raisins instead. Freshly chopped fruit is another useful sweetener, especially pears, melon, bananas or pineapple.

Jam and marmalade are extremely sugary foods, about 70 per cent pure sucrose. As with all sugar, a little does no harm. But there are alternatives – indeed, jam making was only invented about 300 years ago, since before then, there was not enough sugar to make it with. Possible alternatives are honey, peanut butter, yeast extract spread, cheese spread . . . or nothing at all. Good bread tastes fine on its own. You may also like to try making a fruity spread which doesn't contain sugar (see recipes p.29).

Honey is a mixed blessing for the sugar-escaper. It is helpful as a substitute, because although honey contains a high percentage of sugar, it is not sucrose. Almost all the sugar in honey is fructose, or fruit sugar, which has a different effect on the body. Fructose does not cause sudden rises in blood sugar level, because it is much more slowly absorbed through the walls of the digestive passage. It does not stimulate insulin production, so it does not produce sugar's switchback mood effect. On the other hand, eating a lot of honey doesn't help anyone get rid of a sweet tooth. Although it is lower in calories than sugar (80–90 per ounce, compared with 112 per ounce for sugar), you can still get fat on it if you simply swop honey for sugar.

But honey comes in very useful, if you are trying to break a sugar-in-tea or coffee habit. Honey is actually sweeter than sugar, so less needs to be used to obtain sweetness. And because it has its own distinctive taste, the amount of honey you can add to tea or coffee is limited to avoid overpowering the taste of the drink.

So try replacing sugar in drinks with a bare teaspoonful of a mild-flavoured, clear (therefore easy to dissolve) honey, such as clover or acacia.

At main meals desserts are the only real problem. There are different ways of de-sugaring dessert time. The first, and simplest, is to stop making or eating desserts. Instead, you can add a first course to meals if you don't already, or serve larger portions of other courses.

A second alternative is to serve cheese and biscuits and/or fresh fruit for dessert. This is the standard end to a meal in many countries, for example in Eastern Europe, Spain or Italy.

A third option is to make sugar-free desserts. This may be an easier method to start with: especially for those who are dessert fans, or whose family loves them. It is possible to make all kinds of conventional desserts without sugar: baked apples stuffed with dates or other dried fruit; yoghurt with fresh fruit and a little honey; crumble made with honey or treacle instead of sugar; egg custard, using a tablespoonful of honey instead of sugar; fresh fruit salad; dried fruit compote; stewed fruit with sultanas or raisins instead of sugar; milk puddings sweetened by adding dates or raisins before cooking, instead of sugar; and other such adaptations.

Until early 1977, many people may have been happy to use saccharin as a sugar substitute. Now the weight of evidence against this oldest of artificial sweeteners is extremely heavy – see artificial sweeteners in Chapter 4.

Snacks – **sweets, biscuits, cakes, buns, soft drinks and chocolate – are the biggest sugar sources of all.** Our changing meal habits are increasing their popularity. These foods are convenient, easy to obtain wherever you are, relatively cheap, sold in one-person portions, need no preparation, need no cutlery . . . they fit so neatly into a world where more and more meals are eaten quickly, on the move, at offices, and fewer people want to eat at home at mid-day or to go to the trouble of packing lunches. For the same reasons, the sugary snacks are among the hardest foods to avoid. But there are ways of getting round them – once you look for them.

Soft drinks are easy enough to dodge when you are at home. Real fruit juices, home-made lemonade using honey instead of sugar, herb or China tea, milk and other drinks can be used instead. But when you're out, the choice narrows alarmingly. Milk is the one that is easiest to find, but in cafés, tea is often the only alternative to sweet drinks. For office lunches, supermarkets usually sell fruit juice in conveniently small tins and bottles as well as in large sizes. Pub fruit juice is always sweetened, but tomato juice isn't.

Biscuits, cakes, buns and confectionery offer two options: you can substitute entirely different foods, or go to some trouble to obtain sugar-free versions. This usually means making them yourself. Like honey, this option has the advantage of being pleasant to the sweet tooth, and the disadvantage of not helping you get used to not eating sweet foods at all.

Substitutes for sugary snacks which share their appeal of being convenient and sold in one-person sizes include small packets of peanuts and raisins, sandwiches, savoury biscuits, and best of all, fresh fruit. Many people use fruit yoghurt as a snack, not realizing that a small pot can have a sizable amount of sugar in it. Plain yoghurt with fruit added by you is the answer here. For those who can plan ahead, emergency rations of hardboiled eggs, small pieces of cheese, raw carrots, celery, almonds, bread or fruit are all easy to carry from home, as a talisman against the empty calorie offerings of station buffets or school tuckshops.

Step 5. Take another sugar count over two or three days. If your average intake per day is now about ¾ ounce, there's no need to cut down any more. Although there's no harm in doing so, as you don't need any unnecessary sugar in your food. If your count reveals that you aren't getting any further, ask yourself why.

The stumbling blocks for many people are emotional and social. Sugary cakes and sweets mean more than food to so many of us. They are connected with childhood, rewards for good behaviour, comfort and security. No wonder we find ourselves turning back to them when our spirits are low.

Once people recognize this emotional tug, they are better able to resist it. Cravings can be seen as such, and transferred to some other, non-sugary treat.

Social situations can be even more tricky. Most of us eat at least a few meals a week with other people, and there's no reason why they should give up sugar if they don't want to. The result can be temptation for the person who is trying to avoid sugar, and even downright pressure from other people to 'give in'. As with vegetarianism (Chapter 5), there sometimes seems to be a social conspiracy to make us all conform to 'normal' eating patterns. Anyone who doesn't attracts an undue amount of attention, which usually takes the form of asking them to justify their different tastes. Why this should be necessary is impossible to argue, for we don't insist that people who dislike bananas say why. Yet there is an unmistakable aggression towards people who eat differently. I'm told people who are giving up cigarettes suffer the same sort of reaction from those around them. Could it be guilt?

How you deal with such reactions will depend on your temperament. The simplest way is probably to joke it off; the least successful, to try to explain in detail just what you are doing. Evangelism is apt to intensify any adverse reaction, and doesn't make for happy mealtimes.

If neither of these pressures applies, and you still can't cut down successfully, try Step 6.

Step 6. The person who finds he just can't cut out or cut down sugar may have to recognize that he is a sugar addict. After all, it isn't like slimming, where one tries to reduce the total amount of food eaten. Here, the only discipline is not to eat one food, leaving dozens of others that can be eaten instead.

If you have to admit that giving up sugar is beyond you by normal means, drastic methods may work. For three or four days, don't eat anything at all except the following: meat, fish, cottage cheese, eggs, salad greens, water/tea/coffee without sugar. You can have as much as you like of these *but nothing else*. This isn't a recipe for healthy living on a long-term basis: it contains hardly any roughage and too much fat and protein. But as these are very filling, they will help you not want to eat anything else. And it seems as though some people's craving for sugar is really a shortage of protein in disguise: enough protein, and they don't want the sugar any more.

Like all eating patterns, eating less sugar is harder to start with, and then becomes routine. It isn't a penance – more an investment in your own well-being.

No-sugar fruit spreads

Apricot spread

4oz dried apricots
1 tbsp honey

Soak apricots overnight in boiling water to cover. Or place in wide-mouthed vacuum flask, cover with boiling water and leave for four hours. When completely soft, purée in a blender or by rubbing through a nylon sieve. Add enough of the water used in soaking to make a thick but workable consistency. Add honey. Pour into jar which has been sterilized with boiling water. Cover tightly, keep in fridge between uses. This makes about 14oz, which will keep for at least a week to ten days. The calorie content is about 22 calories per ounce, compared with about 80 per ounce in ordinary jam or marmalade.

Apple butter

2½lbs sweet apples
8oz honey
½ lemon
1 tsp cinnamon
1 tsp allspice
½ tsp ground cloves

Wash apples thoroughly but do not peel. In large pan, cover barely with water, bring to boil and simmer gently until apples are completely soft and mushy. Purée in blender or by rubbing through nylon sieve. Return pulp to pan, add honey, spices and juice and grated rind of lemon. Simmer very gently, stirring frequently to prevent sticking, until mixture is thick. Pour into hot jars sterilized in boiling water. Cover immediately with airtight seals. Store in cool, dark, dry place. This makes about 3 jars. Calories per ounce about 25.

Summer spread

8oz soft fruit
1 lemon
1 tbsp honey

Mash fruit with fork. Add juice from lemon and honey. Place in sterilized jar. Store in refrigerator where it will keep for three to four days only. Calories per ounce about 10.

FATS

It is difficult to believe that we eat so much more fat than our fellow countrymen of only six or seven generations ago. We are very calorie-conscious, and most of us like to think of what we eat as light and non-greasy. Meanwhile, we tend to picture our forbears' meals as quite the opposite: gargantuan spreads where tables groaned under meat, butter, cream and cheese, pies, hams and game. Such meals existed, but the number of people who had access to them was tiny. Perhaps it was because they were notable that people *did* note them – so that we know of them. For most people, meals were more frugal, and that meant little fat, since fat was relatively expensive.

Fat – animal or vegetable – is now the cheapest source of calories we have, because it is so calorific. And as we have become more prosperous, we have steadily eaten more and more of our calories in this form. The reason why we don't notice doing so is that so much of our food is pre-made. The fat can't be seen. If we had to make every piece of pastry, cake, biscuit, pâté, ice cream and pie from scratch, we'd soon realize how much of them is pure fat.

Fat comprises over one-third of a chocolate bar, about a third of a piece of pastry or pie case, about a quarter of a biscuit or cake, and it is high, too, in things like delicatessen meats and pâtés, where extra fat is added to that already in the meat used. Most people's fat intake adds up to about five ounces a day. Again, does it matter? Until about ten years ago, little importance was attached to the amount of fat we ate. Fat was one of the Cinderellas of nutrition research. It was treated as no more than a useful source of energy. What brought it into the limelight was the realization that heart disease was a major epidemic.

Different names are given to the different events which can trigger off a heart attack, but the overall picture behind coronary artery disease, ischaemic heart disease, coronary thrombosis, or myocardial infarction is similar. The heart is a working muscle, fuelled by nutrients and oxygen, both carried in the bloodstream along the arteries. If enough of the fuel elements are not available, cells of the heart will die, and the heart will cease to function. The reason why the heart is starved of oxygen is that the arteries which carry the blood become clogged up with fatty and fibrous material which sticks to the walls. The final heart attack arises from this gradual build-up which starts in Western man literally from babyhood – yet never starts at all in some people or some nationalities.

The heart attack may be set off by a clot which gets caught in the narrowed artery, preventing blood getting through. Or it may come when exertion increases the heart's activity and its need for extra fuel – which the narrowed artery cannot supply. Or the deposits along the artery walls may become so thick that they one day close the channel completely.

Heart disease is a strictly modern epidemic. It has been recognized for a long time, because post-mortems easily reveal the state of arteries. But until this century, it was so unusual as to be a medical curiosity. Even in 1921, an American doctor recorded seeing his first case of heart disease – after the whole of his training, and two years in practice.

It is because the material which is found in the arteries of heart patients contains a large amount of fat that fat was first suspected of being a cause of heart disease. Since then, cholesterol – the member of the fat family which forms the largest part of the artery-clogging material – has become the ugly sister of the fat family.

But the fact that cholesterol is present in the silted-up arteries doesn't prove that it is eating cholesterol which causes the deposits. For our bodies manufacture cholesterol in addition to what we get from food; and we don't know why, if cholesterol eaten equals cholesterol in the arteries, some people who eat lots of fat get heart disease, but others who eat just as much, don't.

So what do we know? We know that heart disease is not universal. It only occurs among populations who live in 'Western' style. It isn't racial, because people from non-heart disease countries who move to Western countries develop the same risk as natives – if they move as children. 'Western' style living includes a substantially higher intake of fats, particularly animal fats. But although it is an outstanding difference in living styles, it isn't the only one. What about air pollution, treated water, cigarettes, lack of exercise?

We can weed out some living habits, because they've been practised in the West for a long time, longer than we've been dying from heart disease. Since this still leaves quite a number of possibilities we have to ask why nineteen countries with heart disease problems (such as the UK, USA, Scandinavia and New Zealand) decided that the amount of fat people eat does increase their risk of heart disease – and why they recommended that we all eat less fat.

Reason one is that it is clearly established that people who have a low level of cholesterol circulating in their blood are far less likely to have a heart attack. If people change their diet to eat less fat, and especially less animal fat (the only fat that supplies cholesterol), their blood cholesterol level will drop sharply.

Reason two is that studies of certain groups of Western people who for philosophical reasons eat a different diet from most people, which happens to include less fat, show that they have far fewer heart attacks. Seventh Day Adventists, vegetarians and vegans (who eat no animal foods), and Trappist monks all have a much lower than average frequency of heart disease. With the exception of the monks, the rest of these groups share the environment with those who do have heart attacks – suggesting that stress, air and water pollution and the rest are not the decisive factors.

These studies seem to prove conclusively that diet plays an important part, but do they prove that fats are to blame? Not entirely, because the meals these groups eat are different from average in other ways too. They are lower in calories (not surprisingly, for if calorie-packed fats are reduced, it is hard to avoid reducing total calorie consumption), and they also eat more vegetables.

But the lower level of fat is striking, especially since this is one feature of their style of eating which tallies with countries where heart disease is a rarity for anyone. Filipinos, Japanese, rural Africans, Bedouin Arabs – they and other equally far-flung populations eat very different food. But none of them eat much fat.

Reason three is the most obvious of all, although it may not be so important to heart disease as it seems. Fat makes us fat far quicker than anything else, because it is so full of calories. Just look at the non-fatty foods you have to eat to get the amount of calories contained in one tiny, not very filling ounce of fat:

250 calories = 1oz of pure fat (lard or oil) *or* 1¹/₉oz butter or margarine (they contain water too)

OR

4oz bread (about 4 slices)
2½oz breakfast cereal (nothing added)
9oz baked beans
10oz potatoes
⅔ pint milk

two 5oz pots of fruit yoghurt
3 eggs
8oz chicken
8oz cottage cheese
1 lb 2oz apples
1½ lbs plums, broad beans or oranges

You'd find it almost impossible to eat 250 calories worth of foods like green vegetables, root vegetables, tomatoes or soft fruit. You'd have to eat three or more pounds weight of any of them.

Being overweight is a secondary risk factor in heart disease; having heavily larded arteries is the most dangerous condition. Reducing fat consumption tackles both factors. It is also undoubtedly the most effective single measure to take if you want to lose weight. Just because of the concentration, you only have to give up two ounces of food a day – provided it's the fatty part of your food – and you save almost 500 calories. Bronchitis, rheumatism, arthritis and many other common diseases are made worse by overweight.

A new suspicion has recently been levelled at high fat intake: that it is a factor in the development of cancer of the bowel. This is one of the cancers which has been rising steadily this century. It is now the second most common fatal cancer, after lung cancer. Because this cancer is increasing in the West, yet very rare in the same communities who suffer little from heart disease, the same change in living habits has been suspected of being related to both. Those who believe that too much fat contributes to cancer of the bowel link this element of food with fibre, to be discussed later in this chapter.

Action

Heart disease is so common in the Western world, that it is more a question of 'when' than 'if' for most of us. And over half the Western population is at least 8lbs over average, never mind ideal, weight. Reducing fat intake can be done in a similar way to reducing sugar: the first step is to find out exactly how much fat you do eat every day:

Step 1. Keep a record for several days of how much fat you eat. You don't have to weigh portions, but clearly your record will be more accurate if you do.

Step 2. Begin a gradual campaign of substitutions. The

fat-dodging table on pp.36–7 contains some suggestions as to where to start reducing the amount of fatty foods you eat.

What fat intake should you aim for? The 10 per cent of calories people derived from fats in 1800 is a very difficult target, but 15 to 20 per cent is possible. This translates into a little under two ounces of fat per day. You may think that sounds easy – but that is total fat, the fat in eggs, cheese, meat, fish, nuts and milk as well as the sort you can see in butter or oil.

But unlike sugar, you need some fat. Fat performs essential functions in the body, and carries vitamins. The fat-soluble vitamins are A, D, E and K. Animal fats are the best sources of the first two vitamins, vegetable sources richer in the latter two.

Over the last two decades, the importance of vegetable fats for other reasons has been realized. They are the suppliers, the sole suppliers, of one member of the fat family called linoleic acid. This is known as an essential fatty acid (EFA) because the body cannot make it itself. There are also some other important fatty acids in vegetable fats, but these the body probably can convert from other materials, if they aren't supplied in the right form in food. The fats which contain most EFA and related fatty acids are vegetable and seed oils, the richest sources being linseed, wheat germ, safflower, sunflower and corn oil in that order.

It is known that EFAs perform a variety of vital body functions, and details of these are the subject of much research at the moment. But they have reached public attention rapidly for the same reason as cholesterol – heart disease. If cholesterol has become in popular eyes the 'baddy' of the fat family, EFAs have come to be seen as the 'goodies' which can halt or may even reverse the artery-clogging process.

At first it was thought that the vegetable oils rich in EFAs, known as polyunsaturated fats because of their chemical structure, helped lower cholesterol in the blood simply because they were used instead of animal fats. As no vegetable fat contains cholesterol, the body intake of cholesterol was automatically reduced by this 'swop'. But now it is thought that the vegetable fats have an active effect in lowering blood cholesterol, even in someone who doesn't reduce their intake of animal fats at all.

Because most diets which increase the amount of vegetable

fats in the diet also reduce the animal fat intake (and probably total fat intake too), this active cholesterol-lowering effect is hard to show. But while that separation is very interesting, it isn't so important for practical purposes: if we want to reduce the risk of a heart attack, low blood cholesterol will help. Less fat of all kinds, and more of what fat we do eat from vegetable oils, will help achieve that end.

The polyunsaturated fats are also the richest sources of vitamin E – when they are unprocessed. But this vitamin can be affected when oils are processed, either to extract them from the plant, or afterwards in treating them or in making them into margarine. The body's need for this vitamin increases when more polyunsaturated fats are eaten, so it is important to make sure enough vitamin E is obtained.

If the fats are eaten *in* natural food – nuts, seeds, wheat germ – the vitamin is already there. But if they are eaten in processed form, e.g. in refined oils or ice cream, most of it has been lost. That is why cold-pressed oils, extracted from the plant source by mechanical pressure, not by the cheaper methods of heat or solvent extraction, are preferable. You can buy cold-pressed versions of some oils in health food shops. Olive oil is not a very EFA-rich oil, but nor is it like an animal fat. It's fairly neutral.

It is considered that you need about 0.6 milligrams of vitamin E for every gram of polyunsaturated fatty acid. As a typical vegetable oil is 50 per cent polyunsaturated, that means you need about 8.5 milligrams of vitamin E for every ounce of oil you eat.

The vitamin is needed to protect the oils from changing chemically in the presence of oxygen. This is a change to which polyunsaturated oils are susceptible as soon as they are taken from their plant source, and exposed to air. The changes would produce rancidity and new substances which are irritating to our bodies.

Polyunsaturated fats are also being explored in relation to multiple sclerosis. People with this degenerative disease lose the fatty sheaths which normally surround nerve endings, and it is thought that imbalances in or lack of fatty acids may be a contributory factor.

Because of the value to the body of vegetable oils, it is sensible to make them roughly half of all the fats you eat. The most obvious way of doing this is to stop using any animal fat for preparing foods, so that the animal half of your fat comes from built-in fat in meat, fish, cheese, eggs and

Fat-dodging—a typical day *28 grams of fat = 1oz Target for day = 50g*

	Food	*Fat per oz* (grams)	*Trimming the fat*
Breakfast	Milk	1	Use skim milk, which many people can now have delivered; or make up skim milk from powder to use alone or half and half with milk
	Butter or margarine	23 24	Halve amount used by spreading more thinly; or switch to a soft margarine labelled 'high in polyunsaturates'; try USA trick of using cottage cheese as a bread spread
	Egg Bacon Sausage	3 14 9	Eat these foods less often, and instead try cooked breakfasts such as mushrooms or tomatoes on toast, baked beans, or kippers which are mainly unsaturated fat. Low fat breakfast ideas: cereal with skimmed milk, low fat yoghurt with fresh fruit, wholemeal toast with low fat spread, pancakes with fruit
	Cooking fat	28	Just one ounce of this – the kind of dollop people use to cook a fry-up – could use up your whole saturated fat target for a day. Stop cooking in lard or dripping: grill food or poach or boil eggs
Main meals	Beef, lean Chicken Ham and pork Lamb, roast Meat pies	5 2 11 6 6	Avoid fatty meat: see how much higher pork is than others. Grill, roast or casserole instead of frying. Reduce meat portions, but eat more vegetables instead. Try more meals without meat: cauliflower cheese, bean dishes, etc. Read a vegetarian cookbook for ideas – there are literally hundreds
	Chips	2½	A real fat-food. Eat your potatoes baked, boiled, mashed instead
	Fish, fried Fish, oily e.g. herring, tuna, kipper	3 4	White fish is almost fat-free – use freely. Grill or bake fish; the fat in fish is much less saturated than meat fat
	Cheese, hard Cream, double Cream, single	10 13½ 6	Think of cheese as an alternative to meat, not to eat at same meal. Double cream is so high in fat, it is best avoided completely except for special occasions. Keep for meatless meals
	Pastry	10	Pastry is one-third hidden fat, and very high in calories therefore too. Try to

	—plain	4	
	Cake, fruit	4	Make your own cakes with oil or soft margarine – but using less fat in total
	—rich sponge	7	
	Chocolate	10	Try some alternative snacks to chocolate, crisps and ice cream, which are always very high in saturated fat. Peanuts are high in fat too, but it is unsaturated
	Ice cream	3	
	Crisps	10	
	Peanuts	14	
Snack suggestions			* fresh fruit * low fat yoghurt with fruit or honey * raw carrots, tomatoes, celery or other vegetables * plain biscuits, or your own made with oil or soft margarine * crispbread with cottage cheese, yeast extract and salad topping * a handful of almonds, hazel nuts or walnuts and raisins * dried apricots (very sweet), figs or prunes * wholewheat bread with cottage cheese and salad topping * an ounce of breakfast cereal, moistened with fruit juice
Low fat main meals	*Appetizers*		* thin soups or vegetable soups free from cream * sea food salad or cocktail, without dressing * melon * grapefruit * asparagus, with vinaigrette, not mayonnaise * fruit juices * sea food * corn on the cob, without butter
	Entrées		* all fish * stuffed vegetables, without creamy sauces * pasta dishes, without hard cheese * rice dishes: paella, risotto, chop suey etc * bean dishes, from baked beans to pease pudding * baked potatoes with toppings other than cheese and butter * vegetable casseroles
	Desserts		* fruit or fruit salad * sorbets * pancakes * recipes where hard fats are replaced by oils or soft margarine

milk. The vegetable fats will come from oils for cooking and salads (cold pressed being best), from margarine*, and from nuts and peanuts. There's also a substantial amount of fat in wheat germ and avocado pears.

The biggest problem in reducing fat consumption is the 'hidden' fats. Most of these are also the animal, hard fats of which we need little. Pastry, chocolate, cakes, cream, potato crisps and snacks, sweets like fudge, biscuits and ice cream are the biggest fat-carriers. This doesn't mean that you can't

Fat in food

Only animal and dairy foods contain cholesterol. However, since the link between cholesterol and heart disease is far less certain than the link between hard, animal fats and heart disease, it is simplest to ignore cholesterol, and just reduce total fat intake. Keep animal fat grams to about half daily total.

But you need not calculate this exactly nor each day: it does not matter if you eat a lot of animal fat on occasions, provided your general pattern of eating balances this with days when you eat almost none, so that an overall half animal: half vegetable ratio is maintained.

Very low fat foods

The following and related foods are so low in fat, it isn't worth counting:

Beans
Bread
Breakfast cereals, except granola type
Cod and other non-oily fish
Cottage cheese
Egg whites
Fruit – all kinds except avocado pear
Grains, e.g. barley, wheat, maize
Honey
Jam
Milk, skimmed
Pasta
Porridge
Rice
Seafood
Semolina, sago etc.
Soups, thin
Vegetables
Yeast extract
Yoghurt, low fat

* The distinctive characteristic of polyunsaturated fats is softness. Always choose the soft margarines which declare 'high in polyunsaturates'. A label saying 'all vegetable' is not enough, as some vegetable fats are very low in polyunsaturates, and others are saturated to harden them on purpose.

ever eat these, but they must be watched carefully if you want to keep to a 2oz a day limit (see the list of fat in common foods below).

Grams of fat per 28 grams (1oz) of food. All figures for food cooked without added fat:

Food	*Grams of fat*	*Food*	*Grams of fat*
Almonds	15½	Lamb, fat and lean	2
Avocado pear	2½	Liver	2
Bacon, grilled ½ lean	13	Margarine	23
Beef, fat and lean	3	Milk, whole	1
Biscuits, digestive	5½	Oil	28
Brazil nuts	17½	Pastry, shortcrust	9½
Butter	23	Peanuts, peanut butter	15
Cake, sponge	3	Pecan nuts	19
—— rich fruit	4	Pistachios	15
Cashew nuts	12½	Pork, lean	3½
Cheese, cream	14	Potato crisps	10
—— Edam	6½	Pudding, steamed	3
—— hard	8½	Pumpkin seeds	13
—— spread	6	Salad dressing, French ½ oil: ½ vinegar	14
Chicken, lean and fat	½	—— cream	9½
Chocolate	10½	—— mayonnaise	12
Cocoa powder	6½	Salmon, canned	1½
Coconut, desiccated	10	—— fresh	3
Corned beef	4	Sardines, canned	6½
Cream, double	14	Sauce, white	2½
—— single	5	Sausage, average beef and pork	6
—— sour	5	—— continental	6
Crispbread	3	—— liver	6
Duck	2	Sesame seeds	14
Eggs, whole or yolks only	3½	Tuna, canned, with oil	5½
Ham, fat and lean	11	—— drained	2½
—— lean only	3½	Turkey, fat and lean	2
Hazel nuts	10	Walnuts	14½
Herrings	5	Wheat germ	2½
Ice cream	3	Yoghurt, whole milk	1
Kippers	3		

You don't need to go on counting up your fat intake for long: patterns of eating quickly become habit, and much less effort.

But it is worth the effort to start with. Heart disease is now a young person's disease, so this change in living habits can mean not just a year or two of life in old age, but twenty or twenty-five years of extra life in your prime.

FIBRE

As fast as our sugar and fat intake has been rising, our fibre intake has been dropping (see table). Fibre is the structural part of food, related to carbohydrate, but not digested inside the body to provide calories.

It is present *only* in vegetable foods: however stringy and fibrous a piece of stewing steak may seem, it all gets digested. Fibre is highest in foods like peas and beans, root vegetables, cereals which haven't been refined (e.g. wheat grains, wholemeal flour) and the outsides of fruit.

Fibre is now the newest focus of medical attention, so much so that it is almost impossible to read a medical or nutritional journal without the subject coming up at least once. People have known it existed for a long time, and that it was a good treatment for constipation (Kellogg's All-Bran was launched in 1919). But until about ten years ago, nobody looked very closely at what fibre might do inside us, or how it might fit in to the whole picture of human food needs. The reason why fibre wasn't studied was that it wasn't thought of as food, as it doesn't supply calories.

Fibre then and now
Approximate daily consumption of fibre in the USA (grams per person per day)

	1880		*1970*		change in
Starches	food	fibre	food	fibre	fibre intake
Cereals	480	3.2	120	0.3	−90%
Potatoes	300	1.1	120	0.5	−45%
Pulses	60	1.0	60	1.0	no change
Fruit and vegetables	275	2.8	325	3.3	+20%
Total fibre		8.1		5.1	−37%

(Table by Dr. Hugh C. Trowell, from material of Antar et al)

But now we know that fibre, or roughage, does more than 'just go straight through us'. It seems to have an important mechanical, rather than chemical, part to play in keeping our digestive machinery working properly. I say 'seems', because although the need for fibre is now indisputably accepted, we still don't know exactly what it does inside us, or even what it is.

One of the questions still unanswered is whether fibre from vegetables and fruit is as useful to the body as fibre from cereals. Cereal fibre (most common in our diet as bran in wholemeal flour and wholemeal bread) seems to behave like a sponge inside us, mopping up water, and 'wrapping up' the waste products of food in our digestive system in a bulky parcel with fibre and liquid. This parcel is much easier for the intestinal muscles to shift along the digestive canal than a small, dry, hard, quantity of food with little bulk. And when the waste products reach the bowel, the message 'get rid of me' is transmitted more clearly to the nervous system, and executed more easily by the bowel muscles, which have more to get a grip on. This is why cereal fibre acts as a laxative, and why it doesn't usually produce diarrhoea in the process, as purgatives tend to do. It's a mopper-upper of liquid.

Vegetable and fruit fibre, on the other hand, can produce a looseness, and although they certainly have a laxative effect, seem to work differently from the sponge principle. Nevertheless, both kinds of fibre shorten the time that food takes to travel through the body, and it is this property of fibre which is thought to be particularly significant to health.

The doctors who are most interested in fibre are almost all surgeons, and surgeons specializing in intestinal diseases. They are the people who cope every day with gallstones, appendicitis, diverticulitis, ulcerative colitis, and benign and malignant tumours of the bowel. Many such surgeons believe that their patients would not have reached the operating table – and sometimes need not reach it at all – if they ate more fibre. Waste matter can actually get stuck along the digestive passage, and stay there. This is what happens in diverticulosis, a complaint which one person in three over the age of sixty suffers from in Western countries.

The small, hard, dry lumps of waste which a low fibre diet produces require severe contractions of the muscles in the intestinal wall to grip them. These ring-like muscles are supposed to work in sequence, pushing the material along the canal. But if they contract too tightly for too long, the pressure on the walls of the digestive passage in between the muscle rings is enormous. The result is a between-muscle 'blow-out' – in diverticulosis the wall of the digestive system is forced out, forming a little pocket where waste matter sits, and sits, and sits . . .

Some people have these pockets of waste matter for years without them causing any trouble. Others suffer from the excess pressures and contractions in the digestive tube by developing wind, cramps, odd stomach pains and erratic lavatory habits. But in quite a lot of people, the pockets of waste become infected – yes, the food just rots and goes bad – and the result is inflammation and illness which can be fatal. It is a most unappealing disease.

Diverticular (it means 'turning aside') disease is now routinely treated by giving patients bran, and in many cases, this alleviates the symptoms so that the problem never reaches the operating table.

Constipation is a problem that British people alone spend about £15 million a year trying to get rid of with laxatives. Perhaps people are obsessed with their lavatory habits – and perhaps they are right to be.

Constipation does mean that waste products stay a long time inside us. And again, these surgeons argue, that is time when food wastes putrefy and produce harmful bacteria. And a time when toxic substances which the body has sent on its disposal route stay inside us. These surgeons believe that the contact between such poisonous substances and the wall of the bowel is responsible for much illness. The bowel wall is not waterproof, and some of the toxins can cross it and be re-absorbed into the body. They may also encourage the development of cancer of the bowel.

Again, both historical and international evidence supports this theory. Cancer of the bowel, for instance, is increasing steadily in Western diet countries, and its rise coincides with the fall in fibre intake. It is also highest in industrialized areas – but perhaps the toxins wouldn't have the chance to set off a cancerous reaction if the body could dispose of them rapidly. Appendicitis, gallstones and diverticular disease have all shown spectacular increases in Western countries in the last century.

Away from the operating theatre, but still discressing, is a virtual epidemic of 'irritable colon', or mucous colitis. Often diagnosed as 'nerves' and sent away with a prescription for tranquillizers, spastic colon leads sufferers a miserable dance of bloating after meals, constipation alternating with diarrhoea, stomach cramps and feelings of being tied in knots inside. Nerves do often play a part – as symptoms often intensify when people are under stress – but a high fibre diet can work wonders too.

The significant point is that in countries where a diet rich in fibre has produced a fast transit for food through the body – countries where people eat more unrefined grain, pulses and vegetables than we do – these diseases are as unusual as they used to be here. In Africa, for instance, rural communities are almost free from these intestinal 'diseases of civilization' – but in towns where Africans adopt a Westernized diet, the frequency rises even if not quite to Western levels.

If these surgeons are correct in believing that dangerous bacteria are re-absorbed into the body if they are allowed long contact with the bowel wall, low-fibre meals could also be producing other ill-effects almost impossible to trace to them: vague unwellness as the body's balance is disturbed by the presence of toxic substances. But so far, the question of re-absorption is controversial, and with the taboo word 'cancer', menacingly hovering overhead, the theory is unlikely to be accepted by the medical establishment until it is more than thoroughly proved. After all, how determined has the medical world shown itself in discouraging us from smoking – even twenty years after smoking was shown to cause cancer of the lung?

In the meantime, the other benefits of eating more fibre remain. A smoother-working digestive system, with the prospect of it remaining so when all around are losing theirs.

A high-fibre diet has another benefit for the overfed West: it reduces slightly the absorption of calories from food. At Bristol University, Dr K. W. Heaton has shown that people eating a high fibre diet absorbed only about 92½ of every 100 calories they ate. People eating the same amount of low-fibre food absorbed 97 out of every 100 calories. The unabsorbed calories are likely to be calories from fat – Dr Heaton's tests showed that high-fibre eaters excrete more fat. In the next few years, the significance of fibre, fat and transit rates is likely to become much clearer.

Dr Heaton was interested in the role of fibre in the absorption of food. But he was also curious as to whether high-fibre food could help people reduce their food intake.

He asked volunteers to chew their way through 11 ounces of bread. On one occasion they ate white bread, and on another, wholemeal. The white bread eaters got through their ration in 34 minutes; when they ate wholemeal, it took 45 minutes. Moral: high fibre food needs more chewing, and can therefore be useful to anyone who likes eating but doesn't want to eat too much. The food lasts longer! This experiment has been conducted in a less scientific way by dozens of people who change to wholemeal from white bread. 'I find one or two slices is enough, when I used to be able to go on eating the other stuff slice after slice', is the sort of comment I hear.

Action

How much fibre should we eat a day to keep a smooth-working and healthy digestive system? The amount of roughage which produces comfortable and rapid digestion varies with the individual, but from a variety of tests on volunteer groups, half an ounce of bran a day has been established as an amount which works with most people. This is extra to the roughage present in the rest of the food eaten.

This amount of unprocessed wheat bran contributes about 2 grams of crude fibre to the diet. But the notion of 'crude fibre' isn't accepted as adequate nowadays: it means the amount of indigestible material left in food after it has been treated with acids in a laboratory. But there are elements in food which are dissolved by this treatment which would not be dissolved by the digestive process in our bodies. These include some complex carbohydrate structures, such as cellulose, lignins, pectins and pentosans. All of them add up to what is now called 'dietary fibre' – the elements in food which don't give us calories, but are carried through the body, picking up water and so increasing the bulk of waste materials, producing fast and easy transit and elimination.

Unfortunately, up until recently, the only exact analyses of the fibre in food have been of crude fibre. Dietary fibre may be several times as high as the figure for crude fibre. So at present, it isn't possible to give all the exact figures for the dietary fibre in food. But the foods which are high in roughage are known, and tests by Dr Eastwood at Edinburgh University have established the following order among 25 common foods:

Bran
Carrot
Apple
Brussels sprouts
Oatmeal
Aubergine
Spring cabbage
Maize
Orange
Pear
Green bean
Lettuce
Winter cabbage
Peas
Onion
Celery
Cucumber
Broad beans
Tomato
Cauliflower
Banana
Rhubarb
Old potatoes
New potatoes
Turnip

These and similar foods are only fibre-rich if their skins are eaten too – or their outer coatings, in the case of grains like maize. All the members of the pulse family – from processed peas to baked beans – are high in fibre, and so are all the other unrefined grain foods not on this list – brown rice, wholemeal bread containing bran, wholemeal flour for cooking, buckwheat, foods made with oatmeal, and the whole family of seaweed foods, of which agar agar is widely used as a thickener by food manufacturers.

By far the simplest ways of getting your daily fibre are by changing to wholemeal bread, which naturally contains a substantial amount; and by eating a breakfast cereal which either contains bran, or to which you add bran.

When people start increasing their roughage intake they often complain of feeling too full, or perhaps tight round the tummy. This is because of the water-absorbing ability of bran, giving a bulk low-fibre eaters aren't used to. It is a useful feature for those who want to eat less – because there's no doubt that high-fibre foods make you feel full quicker. But it won't last forever. People's insides get used to the new intake of roughage within some weeks, and stop reacting. Some people don't experience the effect at all. If you do, build up your roughage intake slowly – teaspoonful by teaspoonful – over several weeks. Scoffing half an ounce of bran on the first day is asking for trouble as much as eating a couple of pounds of unripe apples!

By the way, there's a campaign to stop calling fibre 'roughage', and start calling it 'smoothage'. Roughage sounds as though it's rough stuff which cleans out your insides rather like a loofah. Smoothage is a much better way of describing the sponge-like, digestion-smoothing effects of bran.

A return to less concentrated foods is a big step towards improving your nutrition, your well-being and your personal 'fuel mix' for energy. And once you become aware of what your eating habits are, in fat, sugar and fibre terms, it isn't difficult to adjust them.

Most of all, it isn't being fussy, or faddy, or narcissistic to bother to change your eating habits to healthier ones. That's a common attitude – but it is your body you are improving and protecting, and only you can decide how much its health is worth to you. We only have one body to last a lifetime, and everything we achieve in life can be helped or hindered by how well our body performs (and looks). Even if all your ambitions are mental ones, the brain is just a collection of cells like the rest of us.

The message is simple: eat as much of your food as possible in a close-to-nature form. Eat your sugar in fruit, your oils in fish or nuts, your bread as whole-grain, and you won't go far wrong. All the unconcentrated foods are there for us to buy – fruit, vegetables, whole grains – all we have to do is choose them. They are the foods we can eat as much as we want of, and not count. Fats and sugars are the foods we want to eat as little as possible of – we'll get plenty without trying. And in between come the foods we need in moderate amounts – protein-rich foods like meat, fish, dairy products and nuts.

3. Preserving the Product

The second big change over the last 200 years is that we now process food *more*. I say more because it would be wrong to say that processed foods are a modern introduction. Cheese, jam and dried fruit are examples of processed foods i.e. the basic ingredients have been changed by man. The difference today is one of degree. **More foods are altered more drastically from their original composition.** But the aim of processing food remains the same as it always was: to make it keep longer. For instance, keeping milk a long time is the prime reason for making cheese. Raisins are simply a method of preserving grapes.

Keeping food a long time is the outstanding characteristic of British food manufacturing today – and of the food manufacturing of every industrial society. The more industrial a country becomes, the longer it keeps food before eating it. So food processing is part of a bigger process: storage. And storage is as specialized an activity as any other industry.

The word 'fresh' has almost lost its meaning when applied to food in Britain today. It has come to mean something akin to 'raw'. But it rarely does mean fresh, because we keep literally every food. The journey from land to plate is a long and complicated one.

Even foods which are not deliberately processed at all, such as greengrocery, must travel the system. A cabbage, for example, is picked one morning, but must wait until a case and then a truckful are picked to make an economical load. The load travels to a wholesale market, perhaps hundreds of miles away. It sits until bought, then journeys on to the greengrocer's shop. Another wait until it is bought, another journey in a shopping bag follow. Once in the buyer's home, our cabbage may be eaten that day, or may wait – up to a week?

Most foods have much longer journeys to make – either directly from overseas, or in steps, with a factory as well as a wholesaler and retailer, between it and our table. Altering food so that it stays edible for as long as possible is a vital step for the food industry to maintain its profitability. The longer the storage and shelf life, the less money lost through having to throw stock away, at every stage of the process.

Storage and processing change food in basic ways, including its nutritional value. The popular concept of processed food 'having all the goodness taken out of it' is nonsense but some important nutrients certainly are lost in processing, and none are ever gained.

There is no easy way of summing up the effects of food processing and storage, because different foods are affected in different ways. Some vitamins and minerals are more fragile and more easily destroyed than others. And because so little is still known about the interaction of different elements in food, it is certain that we do not recognize some of the changes that take place. The loss of a vitamin may, for instance, also diminish the value to the body of the protein in the same food, or block the body's use of another vitamin. We just don't yet know the full details of how food elements depend on each other.

It is easy to write off losses of vitamins and minerals in food processing by saying that they are insignificant for people eating a balanced diet. In my view, this is an irresponsible and arrogant attitude. It assumes that because we do not know what this change in the food means in terms of its total value to the body, it doesn't matter. It assumes that the body is simpler in this respect than we know it is in other ways. It implies that everyone does eat a correctly balanced diet – and that nutrition is not a subject worth teaching or worrying about. In 1976 an article in the British Medical Journal was headed 'Are dietitians a luxury?' It pointed out that the National Health Service employed a total (hardly grand) of about 700 dietitians, but nobody could decide exactly what they should be doing. Most of them work in hospitals, but, says the article, 'much of the traditional work of the hospital dietitian has become obsolete in recent years. No longer are scrupulous dietary regimens prescribed for peptic ulcers, and much of the obsessional attention to detail has gone from the control of diabetics' diets.' Newly qualified dietitians are apparently having difficulty finding jobs – just at a time when the part played by good eating habits in preventing and helping Britain's most rampant diseases is being fully realized.

HOW DOES PROCESSING AFFECT OUR IMPORTANT FOODS?

The order in which I discuss the processing of different basic foods is not meant to indicate their order of importance in the British diet; but perhaps the order in which they occurred to me matches that in which many other people would list their 'basics'. If it does, it may reflect the emotional significance which is certainly attached to foods – and some foods more than others.

But these foods do form between them the major part of most meals in this country. What is done to them, if it affects their nutritional value, is therefore more important than if we ate small amounts of them. Even a minor change in their chemical composition is magnified by the amount of the food eaten. That is why one should be much more aware and cautious about the processing of, for instance, cheese, than of truffles.

I cannot claim to cover every food which is processed. Even less can I describe fully the significance in health terms of all the changes being made to food. For that is the interesting and disquieting area of ignorance: **so far, nobody knows exactly how the alteration of a food's content of one element, say, a vitamin, may also alter its entire character from the body's point of view.** But that such interactions do occur, there can be no doubt. It is well established that many of the nutrients used by the body are interdependent; cases where the body needs one to be able to absorb the other; or where both are essential if the body is to be able to construct a third element we need. Until these interactions are fully understood, we won't know how serious the effect of processing is on our health.

BREAD AND FLOUR

The amount of bread the average person eats has fallen dramatically over the last century. In the Victorian era, bread was the central food in almost every meal for working class people – that is, for most people. Even a generation ago, in 1955, people ate half as much bread again as they do now – about 55oz (3½ lbs) a week, compared with about 36oz (2.2lbs) now.*

*National Food Survey figures

Wheat grain diagram

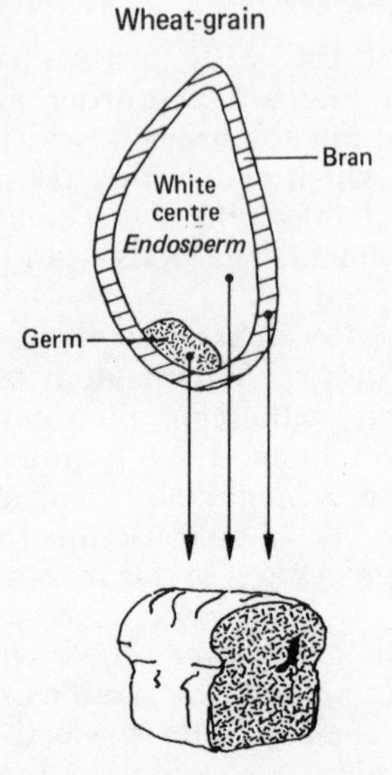

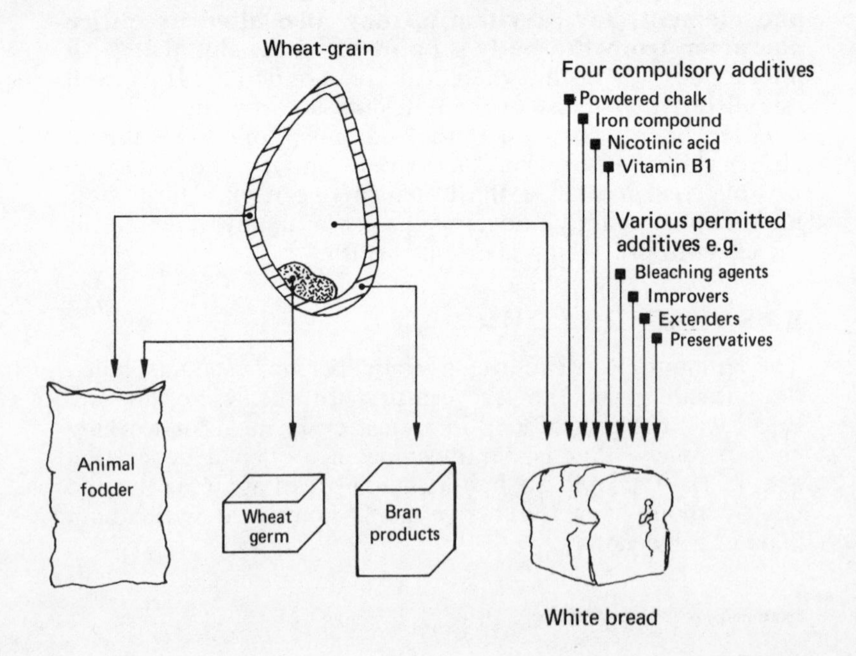

But we still eat very much more bread a week than we do of any other kind of food. The poorer people are, the more bread they eat, together with all the other foods based on flour: pies, pastry, cakes and biscuits. So it is extremely important that flour, on which the food value of all these depends, should be as nutritious as it can be.

White flour isn't. To make it, between 28 and 30 per cent of the wheat grain is removed, and the parts that are removed – the wheat germ and the bran – are far more valuable as foods than the starchy part which is kept. The table (p.52 below) shows how the vitamin, mineral, protein, fat and carbohydrate content of white flour compares with that of wholemeal. The losses are obvious: protein, vitamins, minerals, oils and fibre are lost. Carbohydrates and calories are increased. But the result may be even worse than appears because of the interdependence of food elements. The change of balance during processing towards a mainly carbohydrate food may also have a health significance which we do not yet know.

People often think that this processing only began about 100 years ago, with the introduction of roller flour mills which could separate the different parts of wheat more efficiently than the traditional stonegrinding mills. In fact, some separation of the browner bran and germ parts of the wheat grain from the paler starchy parts has been going on for centuries. The aims were twofold. As always, the main aim of processing was to make the food keep longer. By sieving flour through cloths, it was possible even in medieval times to remove some of the bran and wheat germ. This contains almost all the oils of the wheat grain – oil which can go rancid, spoiling the flour.

The second reason for the sieving was cosmetic. Whiter flour with less bran made finer-textured, higher-rising bread, and was a status symbol. For a long time, richer people ate whiter bread. But by the end of the eighteenth century, almost everyone in Britain was eating bread made from sieved flour.

So pale bread isn't such a recent introduction. But it had nothing like the whiteness we know today, which is due to the rollermills introduced in the 1870s and 80s. Stonegrinding grinds some of the bran and wheat germ up so finely, distributing it through the flour, that no sieve will totally remove it. Rollermilling, in contrast, can 'nick' out the whole of the wheatgerm without crushing it, and remove the several

The food value of white and wholemeal flour compared

	Wholemeal flour	*White flour*
% protein	12	11
% carbohydrate	64.3	72.3
% fat	2.49	1.16
% fibre	2.0	0.12
Vitamins: milligrams per 100 grams		
B1	0.4	0.24
B2	0.12	0.04
Nicotinic acid	5.5	1.6
Minerals: milligrams per 100 grams		
Iron	3.5	1.7
Magnesium	129	22
Calcium	30	142
Manganese	3.4	0.5
Copper	0.625	0.2
Phosphorus	345	92
Potassium	329	93
Sodium	3.3	2.1

The calcium level of white flour is boosted compulsorily by the addition of calcium-carrying chalk to all flour except wholemeal and self-raising. 14oz is added per sack of 280lbs.

The refining of flour also causes the following losses,* shown as percentages of the original amount present in wheat:

Vitamin B6	71.8	Cobalt	88.5
Pantothenic acid	50	Zinc	77.7
Vitamin E	86.3	Selenium	15.9
Chromium	40	Molybdenum	48

Calories Flour contains about 94 calories per ounce when wholemeal; white flour, 100 per ounce. Wholemeal bread: about 65 calories per slice (one fairly thin slice); white bread about 70–72 calories per ounce.

*From Schroeder, H: Losses of vitamins and trace minerals resulting from processing and preservation of foods, *American Journal of Clinical Nutrition*, 24 May 1971.

layers of bran that encase the wheat grain equally cleanly. The diagram (p.54) shows how roller milling works.

By law, millers must add to white flour four of the elements removed in milling: iron, vitamins B1 and B2, and calcium. But they do not have to add back any of the twenty or so other food elements which are removed. Even those four additions are only required in amounts which will match the amounts naturally present in flour milled to 80 per cent (only slightly browner than the 72 per cent of the wheat grain present in white flour). So even with 'fortification', the levels of vitamins and minerals in white flour are considerably lower than those in wholemeal or wholewheat.

There is a further important element the millers would never agree to add back voluntarily: the roughage they have removed from flour with the bran. After all, the second reason for refining flour was to remove this element which produces a rougher-textured, less fluffy loaf. Bran flakes do this by impeding the elastic strands of dough stretching to their maximum height as the dough rises before baking.

Wheat bran is the main source of cereal fibre for people in Britain, and fibre is essential to keep the digestive system working smoothly (see Chapter 2). The arrival of rollermilling meant the virtual disappearance of fibre from white bread. A mere trace remains, rendered even more useless by the fact that we eat much less bread anyway.

At present it is the fibre lost in processing flour that is in the medical limelight. But the other losses – of the wheat germ oil with its vitamin E and polyunsaturated fatty acids, and particularly of many minerals (as shown on the chart) whose role in health is still little understood – may soon seem just as glaring and just as bad. What may take longer to be accepted is the recognition that the *whole* food may be different in nourishment from the total of the different parts of it – that the balance that exists there in nature is a contributor too. If you make a soufflé and leave out the egg whites, you don't just lose some protein and vitamins – the whole thing falls flat!

Crispbreads are an important and new part of many people's diets – and therefore their nutritional value is important too.

Many crispbreads are made from whole grains – such as Ryvita, Macvita and several shops' own brands. They're much better than the others – they have kept their fibre and start out with vitamins and minerals intact.

Roller milling

It is about 100 years since this more efficient method of separating the parts of the wheat grain was developed. Although 'white' flour was produced before by sieving wholemeal, the method of sieving after stonegrinding cannot remove wheat germ oil or all the bran or wheat germ from the flour. The resulting flour was creamy in colour.

This is a much simplified diagram of roller milling. The rolling and sieving is repeated many times.

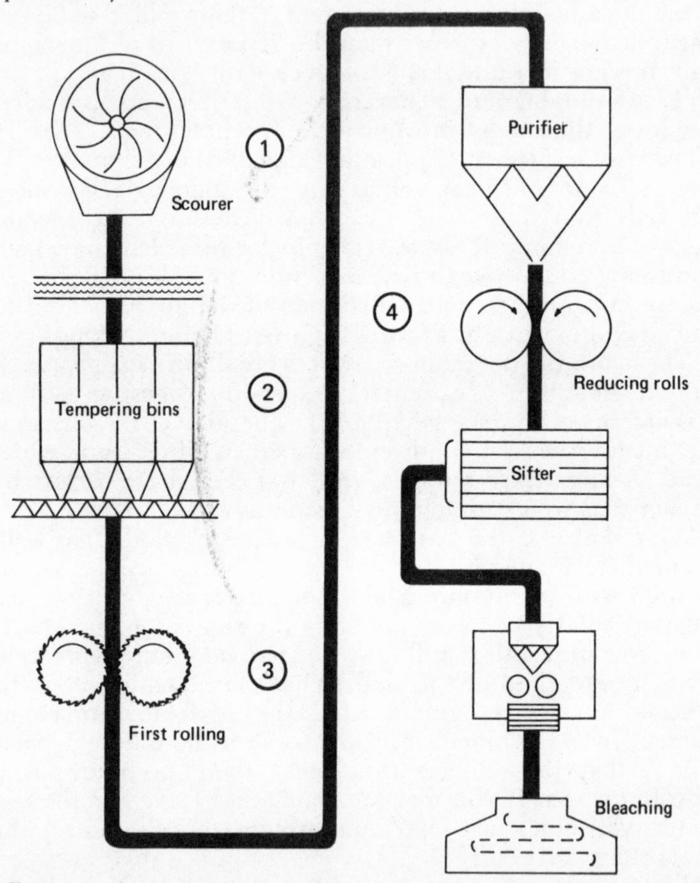

1. *Cleaning*
This cylinder contains beaters which scour impurities and some outer bran coatings from the wheat grain.
It is one of several cleaning stages which stonegrinding and roller mills both use to separate the wheat grains from foreign objects such as other plants, stones or bits of wood.

2. *Tempering*
The water content of the wheat is adjusted to harden the outside of the wheat grain – the bran layers. This makes them more brittle, so they separate more easily from the rest of the grain.

3. *First rolling*
The first set of rollers the wheat grain goes through are corrugated, to break the wheat into large particles.

4. *Sieving and rolling*
The process in this drawing is repeated several times, with different rollers and sieves, to separate the different parts of the wheat grain. The miller ends up with neat piles of bran, wheat germ and endosperm, the starchy part of the grain which is matured and bleached with chemicals for white flour.

But some crispbreads and crackers made from white flour are even less nutritious than white bread. On top of the refining losses, their manufacture involves toasting which means further losses of B vitamins.

Action

Unless you regard yourself as a second class citizen, first class bread is important because, even today, it is the food we eat most of. Lots of people think they eat very little bread, but most of them actually get through quite a lot by the time they've counted sandwiches at lunchtime, snacks, toast, dinner rolls, hot dogs at the cinema, meals out etc.

First class bread from a nutritional point of view is wholemeal. Even if you were getting all the food elements you needed from other foods, you wouldn't be getting much cereal fibre, and wholemeal bread is the easiest way to obtain this.

But buying wholemeal bread isn't as easy as wanting to. On *Here's Health* magazine, we've been testing loaves sold as 'wholemeal' or 'wholewheat' (legally the same) to see if they really are. In a year of spot checks, we've bought over sixty loaves from different towns and different bakers' shops to be analysed for their fibre content. We have often been told 'No, we don't sell wholemeal' and had to try another shop. But finally we've been sold a wholemeal loaf. Not everyone can or wants to hunt – and what they get in the end may not be what they think it is. That's what our fibre tests were testing.

The fibre content you'd expect a wholemeal loaf to have is at least 1.8 per cent by dry weight. Our tests can't prove that a loaf is wholemeal – because a loaf with a high fibre content could be made from white flour with bran added to it. **But they have proved that half of the loaves we've tested haven't been wholemeal, because their fibre content was too low.** We've bought the loaves as ordinary members of the public, and they've been tested by an independent analyst – and it looks as though half the bread sold by bakers' shops as wholemeal is a con. Sometimes it is nearly wholemeal, sometimes its fibre content is so low that it looks like white flour to which caramel has been added. It's quite legal, by the way, to colour brown or wholemeal bread with caramel.

But it isn't legal or honest to say a loaf is wholemeal when it isn't. *Here's Health* has been trying to make people aware that it is no use going and asking for 'brown' bread, or taking wheatmeal as wholemeal. It never is. 'Don't say brown, say wholemeal' is the slogan we'd like to adapt from that other slogan!

You can get genuine wholemeal bread from many bakers, if you insist. It's often not a deliberate confusion on the baker's part, for shop assistants sometimes don't know wheatmeal from wholemeal. You can get wholemeal bread more easily from health food shops – where they make an effort to have it made without additives too. If you can, find such a shop, or better still, bake your own wholemeal. Then you can guarantee its contents.

I'm still amazed how many people are fascinated yet frightened by the idea of breadmaking. I'm still being told how clever I am to make my own – and how they'd love to, only they don't have the time. Well, I reckon I have less free time than lots of people. But I think that anyone who uses lack of time as an excuse doesn't really want to make bread: **if you have time to care about the quality of your life, you've time to make bread.** Because it doesn't take long. As it happens, I'm making bread while I'm writing this chapter. It keeps quite well, so I make it about once a week, except when I have guests. The only bread I buy is in emergencies, or loaves for the analyst!

I use four ways of making bread, according to how much time I have. The longest takes 95 minutes start to finish, of which 15 minutes involve my presence. The shortest takes 40 minutes, with 1 minute flat of effort for me. Here they are:

(1) 95 minutes

3lb wholemeal flour
1oz dried yeast/2oz fresh
1oz sea salt
1oz fat (any kind – oil or butter – important to delay staling)
½oz sugar (any kind)
1 vitamin C/ascorbic acid tablet – 50mg strength
1½ pints warm water

Measure the water: the easiest way to get the right temperature is to mix one pint cold and half a pint boiling water. Put half a pint of water and the vitamin C tablet in a bowl. Add 1 teaspoon of the sugar and the yeast. If using dried yeast, you now leave it time to 'come back to life' in these favourable surroundings – warm, wet and with some sugar to feed on. Cover and leave in a warm, not hot, place for about 10 minutes until it has a head on it like a glass of stout. Add your fresh yeast or frothy dried yeast mixture to the rest of the warm water and tip the whole lot on to your flour, salt, fat and remaining sugar. Mix with a spoon or your hand, and when a dough has formed, tip on to a floured surface for kneading.

This is where the vitamin C comes in – I don't just add it for fun. Vitamin C is added to about three quarters of commercially made bread nowadays. A clever Dr Chamberlain, working at the Flour Millers and Bakers Research Association, developed a method for bread making where the baker used a high speed mixer to mix the dough. He found that this and the addition of certain acids helped the dough develop more quickly the structure that it needs to have before baking. Ascorbic acid, or vitamin C, as we familiarly know it, was chosen because nobody would object to it as an additive. Because the Millers research station is at Chorleywood, the process was christened the Chorleywood Bread Process. It's now used for 75 per cent of UK bread. The advantage of this method for the baker is that it eliminates the need for the dough to sit and ferment whilst this dough structure develops slowly over several hours. That calls for bakers to get up early and mix the dough to start with. With the new method, bakers can get up later – and so can housewives.

Knead the dough for 6–10 minutes, and you'll find that in the middle, it changes its texture, and becomes silkier and smoother. Now cover it with a polythene bag or damp cloth, just while you warm and grease bread tins. This recipe makes four 1 lb loaves, fancy loaves or what you will. I find tin loaves the most practical for making toast, sandwiches for packed lunches and storage. Divide the dough into pieces. Each 1 lb loaf needs about 18oz of dough – you lose about 2oz of water during baking. Standard small shop loaves, by the way, weigh 14oz. Knead each piece for a few seconds, then flatten it with your palm, and turn the edges to the middle to make a sausage shape as long as the tin. Turn it over and drop into the tin with the smooth side upwards.

That's the end of the work part. Now cover the tins with polythene, and put in a warm place (airing cupboard, on top of stove, or on top of a pan of simmering water). Leave for about 30 minutes until dough has risen just above the top of the tins. Meanwhile, heat the oven to maximum temperature. The dough's rising time will depend on room temperature. Even in a cold room, it will rise eventually, but it will take hours. That's why warming the tins and water is important. Never be tempted to let bread rise too high – if you do, its stretch may be exhausted and it may collapse in the oven. If you find it's over-risen while you didn't notice, you can always re-knead for a minute to knock the air out, and let it rise again (which it will do even quicker).

Put in a hot oven, turning the temperature down after 5 minutes to 425°F, 210°C, gas mark 7. Bake for a further 30 minutes. The cooked loaf should sound hollow when tapped – and shouldn't hiss as it does while baking. Remove from tins immediately and let cool.

Overnight method This is the same 95-minute recipe, adapted for when it's late at night and I need bread tomorrow, but want to go to bed. I mix the dough with slightly cooler water, knead and put into cold greased tins. Then I put them in the 'fridge and go to bed. In the morning, the first thing I do is heat the oven. The bread will have risen. I transfer it straight from the 'fridge to oven and bake as usual. If I let it sit in the warm room while the oven heats, it may rise too far.

(2) No-knead 80-minute recipe

This is slightly quicker than my ordinary recipe, and I use it when I'm just feeling lazy. It is better known as the Grant loaf because the method was publicized by Doris Grant, author of *Your Daily Bread* and lifelong campaigner for wholemeal bread as part of a natural food diet. This method produces a very different kind of loaf – because much more water is used. I have heard it described by a master baker as 'waterlogged', and I suppose that that is true. However, we like the texture, which has lots of little holes. It keeps well.

The ingredients are just the same as for ordinary bread, but you add your yeast mixture to the other ingredients and then add as much more warm water as you need to obtain a stiff, just-stirrable dough. I can't give an exact amount, because flours differ in their absorbency, but the dough should be just too wet to knead, although much thicker than a batter. Give it 50 stirs with a wooden spoon, then transfer (it won't really pour) into warmed, greased tins, filling them about half full. Cover and leave to rise for 30 minutes, pre-heating the oven in the usual way. Then bake, turning heat down to 400°F, 200°C, gas mark 6 after a few minutes. Baking time is about 35 minutes. The loaf won't sound hollow (too much water) but if you want to check, pierce with a warm skewer, which should come out dry.

(3) 40 minute soda bread

Soda bread doesn't appeal to everyone, but it is very good in-a-hurry bread. You lose about 10 per cent more B1 vitamin by using soda, and if you don't measure the soda carefully, you get a nasty taste from it. Too much soda can irritate your stomach, but the right amount should disappear in the baked bread: it should all react with the acid of the sour milk in the bread to give off gas which forces the bread to rise. Of course, you gain some food value too, from the milk.

1 lb wholemeal plain flour
½ pint sour milk
1 oz fat or oil
1 teaspoon salt
1 large teaspoon bicarbonate of soda

Pre-heat the oven to 425°F, 210°C, gas mark 7. If you don't have any sour milk, or buttermilk which does just as well, warm milk with a tablespoon of lemon juice to make it sour. Sift flour, soda and salt, rub in fat. Grease baking sheet or large loaf or cake tin. Tip liquid on the flour, mix quickly and knead in bowl for about half a minute, just until smooth. Put into greased tin, or onto baking sheet where it should be deeply scored with a knife (which helps it rise). Bake immediately for 30–35 minutes. Cool away from tin.

A final way of speeding up the basic wholemeal recipe is to make rolls instead of loaves. These only need 'proving' – leaving to rise – for about 15 minutes, and 10–15 minutes baking.

You can do all your home baking with wholemeal flour – with the exceptions of flaky and puff pastry. **Most people seem to think that wholemeal is only for bread, but it can be used just as well for pastry, buns, cakes and biscuits.*** The results will be different from using white flour. Cakes will rise less, for instance, but they will have a good texture in their own way; at first, people find it hard to break away from the brainwashing they've received as to what the things they bake should look like. But after a while, you'll probably find that white cakes and biscuits seem

*See *The Wholemeal Kitchen*, M. Polunin et al (1977)

unsatisfying and 'all air', without the flavour and nuttiness that wholemeal flour adds. Because of the difficulty of buying ready-made foods made with wholemeal flour, baking your own pastries and biscuits is really even more important than it is with bread, which can be found.

You don't need a special recipe book to bake with wholemeal, although you may find one encouraging. You can simply adapt ordinary recipes. Change the flour from white to wholemeal – and perhaps use a little more liquid in the recipe, as wholemeal is more absorbent.

VEGETABLES AND FRUIT

The greengrocer is the last bastion of fresh food in an industrial society. And he is besieged! Year by year, frozen, dehydrated and canned vegetables and fruit conquer more of the market.

Large-scale catering, whether in schools, hospitals, work canteens, the Forces or big restaurants, has almost completely abandoned fresh vegetables and fruit. They consider them too expensive in terms of the labour needed to prepare them, wastage because they are perishable, effort needed to buy them and care to cook them. If they do use fresh ingredients, they tend to abuse them . . . of which more later.

Unfortunately, processed vegetables of all kinds are very inferior in nutritional value to fresh ones. The reasons can be crystallized in one word: 'fragility'. While some foods are so composed that their nutritional value stands up well to processing (and can even be enhanced), the goodness in fresh vegetables and fruit is of an easily destroyed nature. It is at its height when the vegetables or fruit are growing in the ground. The minute – yes, literally the minute – they are harvested, the elements of value to man begin to decline.

The main nutritional value of produce is vitamins, minerals, carbohydrates and sugars, and fibre. Vegetables contribute more vitamins, in general, than fruit. Most of the vitamins present are either part of the B group, or vitamin C. This means that they will dissolve in water, and are sensitive to heat, to light and to contact with oxygen, i.e. air. Now consider the obstacle course these vitamins have to run in processing. Although manufacturers may go to impressive lengths to speed the harvested vegetables to the processing plant, all preserving methods involve peeling – perhaps aided by hot steam or chemical solutions – in which exposure to air and heat begin to whittle away the vitamin content as quickly as the peeling process itself does. Important fibre is also lost here. Chopping, dicing or slicing all increase the surface area exposed to destructive oxygen-reaction (oxidation). Any soaking will carry away in the water both vitamins and mineral salts.

Now for the specific process: in freezing, canning or drying, vegetables are first blanched – dipped for perhaps a minute or two into boiling water – in order to inactivate enzymes, protein-type substances in every live thing, which act as the organism's tools for breaking down and using chemical structures. Unfortunately, enzymes have what one might call a destructive nature . . . and in produce this leads them to start breaking down the structure of the plant as soon as it is plucked from its natural habitat. Enzymes will destroy vitamins and change the texture and colour of vegetables and fruit. So isn't inactivating them with heat a good thing? In the context of food processing, it is certainly a necessary step, if the nature and colour of the produce is to be preserved. But the exposure to heat and water in blanching destroys vitamins too. And enzymes themselves may have a value to man – although they are little understood yet.

After blanching, produce may be treated with a preservative such as sulphur dioxide. This is to slow down the reaction with oxygen which would normally result in browning – something we've all seen when we cut an apple or banana. Sulphur dioxide (see Chapter 4) also prevents any micro-organisms in the food developing and spoiling it. Again, a necessary step, and one which helps preserve vitamin C content. But sulphur dioxide effectively destroys vitamin B1.

Drying exposes produce to a further loss of goodness through more contact with air: left to proceed, it would cause rancidity of any fats in the foods. Although we think of vegetables and fruit as fat-free, almost every food contains some fat, and vegetables do after all supply oil. To avoid rancidity, which would spoil the taste of the dried vegetable or fruit, and which would also produce harmful irritants to the person eating them, antioxidants may be added (see Chapter 4).

Drying vegetables and fruit is probably the most vitamin-destructive form of preservation – and some minerals and

The essential vitamins

Vitamin	*Best food sources*	*Function*	*Deficiency signs*	*Minimum daily need*
A **retinol**	Fish liver oil, oily fish, liver, kidney, dairy foods, margarine, green vegetables, yellow fruit	Essential for growth, health of eyes, structure and health of skin	Low resistance to infection, night blindness, catarrhal and bronchial infections, skin complaints	Children under 13: 1200iu (= 360mcg). Adults: 2500iu (= 750mcg)
B1 **thiamin**	Yeast, wheat germ, meat, soya beans, whole grain foods, green vegetables	Essential for growth, conversion of carbohydrates into energy, health of nerves, muscles	Nervous disorders, skin and hair disorders, depression, poor digestion	Children under 13: 0.8mg Adults: 1 – 1.2mg
B2 **riboflavin**	Yeast, wheat germ, meat, soya beans, eggs, vegetables	Essential for growth, health of skin, mouth, eyes, general well-being	Dry hair and skin, mouth sores, nervousness, lack of stamina	Children under 13: 0.8mg Adults: 1.7mg
pantothenic acid	Yeast, liver, wholemeal bread, brown rice, eggs	Health of skin and hair, including hair growth. Needed for all tissue growth	Dry skin and hair	Children under 13: 2.5mg Adults: 5 – 10mg
B6 **pyridoxine**	Yeast, wheat germ, meat, fish, wholemeal products, milk, cabbage	Essential for body's use of protein, health of skin, nerves and muscle	Irritability, depression, skin eruptions, insomnia, muscle cramps	2mg. Women taking oral contraceptives need much more
B12 **cobalamins or cyanocobalamin**	Liver and meat, spinach, eggs, lettuce	Health of nerves and skin, body's use of protein, growth	Anaemia, tiredness, skin disorders	Children under 13: 0.5 – 1mcg Adults: 1 – 5mcg
biotin	Liver, kidney,	Probably essential for	Falling hair, eczema	Children under 13:

(B group)		prevent build-up of fats in body	tolerance	Adults: 10mg of each
folic acid (B group)	Offal meats, green vegetables, yeast	Essential for all growth, healthy blood, fertility	Anaemia, weakness, depression, diarrhoea	0.5mg
niacin nicotinic acid (B group)	Fish, poultry, yeast, peanuts	Essential for growth, health of skin, digestion of carbohydrates, nervous system	Skin disorders, nervous and intestinal upset, headaches, insomnia	Children under 13: 5 – 16mg Adults: 18mg
C ascorbic acid	Citrus fruit, other fruit, raw vegetables	Essential to health of cells, blood vessels, gums and teeth, healing of wounds	Sore gums, low resistance to infection, slow healing, painful joints	30mg is minimum
D calciferol	Fish liver oils, sunshine on skin, oily fish, butter and margarine, eggs	Formation of bones and teeth, needed for calcium and phosphorus use	Retarded growth, crooked bones (rickets), tooth decay, weak muscles	Children under 13: 250iu (= 10mcg) Adults: 100iu (= 2.5mcg)
E tocopherol	Vegetable oils, wheat germ, wholemeal bread, egg yolks, green vegetables, nuts	Known to be essential, but function not fully understood. Needed for fertility and muscle health by animals	In animals, muscular disorders, infertility and nervous disorders	Not certain but estimate at 10iu (= 10mg)
K	Green vegetables, soya beans, liver, oils	Essential for blood clotting	Prolonged bleeding from cuts or sores	About 100mcg

fibre are lost too. Yet it is a growing method, with dried produce forming the basis of packet soups, dessert mixes and millions of catering meals a week. It's so convenient – the packets keep forever. It's cheap to transport because it's light. That 'proof that there is intelligent life on earth' – instant mashed potato – has alone and in a single decade, removed from British meals literally tons of vitamin C – of which potatoes are normally the single main contributor. Mashed dried potato has had every vestige of its original vitamin C destroyed.

If blanched vegetables are destined to be tinned, they must next be cooked. It is truly amazing that people fail to realize that *anything* canned is cooked . . . whether it is cream or cabbages. Heating in the tin is *why* tinned food does not go bad. Cooking means heat, so more vitamins are lost; and it usually means water-contact too, so that a further proportion of vitamins and minerals will transfer from food to surrounding liquid. Whether this is a loss depends on whether we drink the liquid, as in soup (no loss) or throw it away (canned potatoes). Canned vegetables and fruit are often a mainstay of diet for the least well-off and worst nourished part of the community who can also least afford these losses of goodness. And of course, they dominate catering.

In comparison with drying and tinning, freezing seems positively virtuous in nutritional terms. This newest and fastest growing method of preserving also involves blanching produce, but the other losses are avoided. The cold temperature inactivates enzymes and micro-organisms, so no preservative or cooking is needed.

But all processed produce undergoes one more loss that is almost ignored. Neither freezing, canning nor drying suspends animation entirely. Losses of vitamins continue, little by little, as a tin or packet sits on a shop and then a household shelf, or as frozen foods nestle in the supermarket or domestic freezer.

Manufactures of processed foods often defend their products by comparing their carefully timed, expert processing of vegetables and fruit with the less controlled treatment they are likely to receive at home. Frozen can be better than fresh, they say. And of course, they have a good point. When dealing with fresh vegetables, a domestic cook can destroy vitamins and minerals with at least as much ruthlessness as a canning machine. It is only the household cook, after all, who lets the cabbage boil on because the telephone rang.

And to return to the catering scene, an establishment catering for hundreds of lunches will pre-peel, pre-soak, pre-chop, pre-cook and keep warm vegetables in a way that would make any commercial canner blush.

But what the processors ignore is that some of this destruction will be applied to processed produce too. It will be piled on top of the losses of goodness that have already taken place. Canned, dried or frozen produce will be heated again. Its vitamins and minerals, if there are any left, will have to run another gauntlet of heat, water and air before they are eaten.

Action

Forget about processed fruit and vegetables. Remind yourself that your great grandmother got on all right without them, and she didn't have the marvellous choice of fresh produce we have today. **Without our support, the greengrocer will disappear. Fresh vegetables are still one of the cheapest foods around, and if we treat them gently, the most nutritious.**

Everyone should be taught at school the golden rules of looking after vegetables and fruit. Here are mine:

1. Only buy fresh fruit and vegetables.
2. Keep them as short a time as possible.
3. Store them in the dark in a cold place. The bottom of the fridge is ideal.
4. Don't get vegetables ready hours in advance: only expose them to air or liquid for the minimum time. No pre-soaking, pre-peeling, pre-chopping. Where possible don't peel them at all.
5. Cook vegetables for as short a time as possible, in as little liquid as possible.
6. Eat as many as you can without cooking them at all.

BREAKFAST CEREALS

The latest survey, Kelloggs Breakfast Survey, 1977, shows that breakfast cereals are playing a bigger and bigger part in the British diet. Forty per cent of Britons now base their breakfast on cereal, which is twice as many as a mere twenty years ago when a similar survey was done. That's besides all the people who eat cereal with a cooked breakfast. The younger you are, the more likely it is that cereals form a substantial proportion of your total food. Children often eat cereals as an evening meal as well as at breakfast, and in more and more households, the convenience of cereals is used by parents who let their children help themselves to breakfast.

So the processing of cereals is important. It is ironic that cornflakes, the first breakfast cereal (apart from oats for porridge) was invented in the 1880s as a health food. The pioneer was Dr John Kellogg, a Seventh Day Adventist who had a sanitarium at Battle Creek, Michigan. Dr Kellogg thought he was producing a 'basic' food to add to the natural food régime which he used with great benefit on patients, many of whom were suffering from a surfeit of rich cooking. Cornflakes are made by cooking refined maize to a gruel, which is shaped into flakes which are then baked crisp.

So what is wrong with that? The answer is: overprocessing. First, the processing of the grain. The grains on which cornflakes and dozens of other cereals which followed them are based are wheat, rice and maize. In their natural state, these are sources of a variety of important food elements: the table below shows some of them. In addition to these, small amounts of many minerals which are essential to man are present.

The situation is very different after refining – where the 'germ' – the part of a grain from which a new plant would grow – and the outer bran layers, are removed. The refined grain has less protein, less B vitamins, hardly any of the plant oil which is rich in polyunsaturated, essential fatty acids – the sort man can't make himself. The loss of oil also means loss of vitamin E. Refined grain is lower in minerals and very low indeed in fibre. Breakfast cereals based on refined grains include cornflakes, Rice Krispies, Special K, and all the sugared, chocolate-flavoured versions of these.

But not all cereals are made from refined grain – as the advertisements point out, wheat biscuits, puffed wheat and puffed rice and shredded wheat cereals are based on whole grains. So aren't they as good as the whole grain itself? No, because the second step in making cereals – the physical re-shaping of the grain into the desired form – is also very vitamin-destructive.

The cereals based on unrefined cereals are better because they keep their bran and germ – avoiding the first losses listed above. But the extremes of heat and exposure to air and light involved in flaking, puffing, shredding, toasting,

Cereals: food value of wholegrain v. refined (per 33 grams – just over one ounce, equivalent to the weight of an average serving of breakfast cereal, without milk or sugar added)

	Maize		*Rice*		*Wheat*	
	whole	*corn-flakes*	*whole*	*puffed*	*whole*	*flakes*
Calories	120	120	118	113	113	125
Protein (grams)	3.1	2	2.7	2	3–5a	3
Fat (grams)	1.5	0.3	0.5	0.3	0.7	0.7
Vitamin B1 (milligrams)	0.1	0.01	0.08	0.03	0.1	trace
Vitamin B2 (milligrams)	0.04	0.01	0.02	trace	0.05	0.01
Vitamin B6		–	0.5	–	0.1	–
Vitamin B group:						
Pantothenic acid (milligrams)		–	0.4	–	0.5	–
Vitamin E (milligrams)		0.04	0.7	–	0.3	0.1
Calcium (milligrams)	4	2.5	3.3	1.3	13	6
Iron (milligrams)	0.8	0.4	0.6	0.25	1	1
Magnesium (milligrams)		5	45	13	33	–
Fibre	0.5	trace	0.3	0.3	3.5	3.5

(a: protein content of wheat varies widely according to source and variety; USA and Canadian wheats normally contain the higher amount)

and pre-cooking break down most of the B vitamins, and may also change the usefulness of the food to the body in other ways we don't appreciate. But the losses we can appreciate are quite enough – as is clear from the comparison of wholegrain and refined versions in the table above.

These kinds of breakfast cereals are just not good foods – a fact recognized by some of their manufacturers in adding extra vitamins to some products. The vitamins added back are usually some of the B group – B1, B2 and niacin. But these are only three of the many vitamins in whole grains. Nothing is done to restore the others, or the minerals lost in the kinds based on refined grains. Nor do all manufacturers do some 'adding back'. Some maintain that their products have a nutritional value in that they are a vehicle for drinking milk and adding sugar; others see their products as 'fun foods' whose nutritional deficiencies are not important because, they argue, people make up on the other foods they eat.

There are breakfast cereals which pass on to the eater the same value as the unprocessed, whole grain: oats, for

Food value of porridge made with water, not counting added milk or sugar

	Porridge made from 1oz oats
Calories	110
Protein (grams)	3.3
Fat (grams)	2.2
Vitamin B1 (milligrams)	1.4
Vitamin B2 (milligrams)	0.03
Biotin (micrograms)	5.5
Vitamin B6 (milligrams)	0.03
Pantothenic acid (milligrams)	0.25
Vitamin E (milligrams)	0.45
Calcium (milligrams)	16.5
Iron (milligrams)	1.1
Magnesium (milligrams)	33
Fibre (grams)	0.4

instance, whether eaten as porridge or uncooked in muesli. Muesli, or 'Swiss breakfast cereal', is another way of obtaining the same, unrefined, food values. But there is a snag here – the amount of sugar that many commercial mueslis contain. Adding sugar adds nothing but empty calories to muesli: and dilutes the goodness of the other ingredients. Dried fruit, and chopped nuts, are better additions: both provide vitamins and minerals, the nuts also add valuable oils and protein.

The original muesli recipe was developed by Dr Bircher-Benner for his clinic near Zürich. Unlike Dr Kellogg, he ended up with a truly nutritious dish. But it has been bastardized by many, although not all, commercial versions. The original muesli was intended as a whole meal, not as a breakfast course. The serving of cereal was one tablespoon per person only, not a bowlful! To that cereal was to be added lots of fresh fruit – a large grated apple, fresh lemon juice, freshly chopped nuts and cream, yoghurt or milk to moisten. No sugar! People today complain that muesli is fattening. The cereal + sugar + milk version is. Dr Bircher-Benner's fruity meal isn't.

Wheatgerm and bran can be used as breakfast cereals – although most people only find them enjoyable eaten with something else, such as fruit or muesli. Because they are extracted from the wheat grain, you can't really call them 'whole foods', but added to wholewheat, they certainly pack a lot of vitamins and minerals into your cereal. See how much on p.70 – and also what you lose when they are taken away in grain or flour refining. The protein level in wheatgerm, for instance, is higher than in meat, and provided it is eaten with other foods, as valuable.

Wheat germ is the richest source of Vitamin E in common foods. Unfortunately, it also carries with it the problem of rancidity. Most wheat germ, e.g. Froment, Bemax and other brands, is stabilized – a heat process which inactivates an enzyme which would otherwise make the germ vulnerable to rancidity. Stabilization is another piece of processing, but it's definitely better to eat stabilized wheat germ than rancid wheat germ (it should say whether it's stabilized or not on the packet). If you prefer, as I do, the unstabilized kind, only buy a little at a time and from a shop with a brisk turnover. Keep it in an airtight container in the refrigerator. Use within three weeks – a good incentive to eat it regularly! Stabilized wheat germ keeps for a few months.

What about bran cereals? At the present time, fibre is still a rather mysterious component of food. We know we need it, but a lot of work still has to be done to establish how its value to us can be affected by the form we get it in. It is known that bran in large particles has more effect in 'hurrying up' the digestive system than fine ground bran. And that cereal fibre has a different effect on us from vegetable fibre. But the relative value of cooked versus uncooked bran has not been established. Even measuring fibre is still controversial. So we can't say whether bran cereals are as good for us as uncooked bran.

Food value per ounce

	Wheat germ	*Bran*
Calories	105	62
Protein (grams)	8.5	4.6
Fat (grams)	2.5	1.3
Vitamin B1 (milligrams)	0.45	0.2
Vitamin B2 (milligrams)	0.2	0.1
Biotin (micrograms)	–	–
Vitamin B6 (milligrams)	–	0.44
Pantothenic acid (milligrams)	–	0.7
Vitamin E (milligrams)	7.3	–
Calcium (milligrams)	20	34.5*
Iron (milligrams)	22.5	4.3*
Magnesium (milligrams)	0.9	142
Fibre (grams)		10

*the calcium and iron in bran are not as useful as they look: the body absorbs them very inefficiently from bran because of the form in which they are present

Bran cereals have lost some B vitamins in the process of being formed into flakes or other shapes. But they are still superior nutritionally to other cereals, because most people need some extra roughage to offset the lack of it in the rest of their food, and because bran starts out being a better source of vitamins, minerals and protein than refined cereals. Also, most bran cereals have less added sugar than many cereals.

Action

A breakfast cereal can be just as good a breakfast as a cooked meal. But only if you pick the cereal. **Avoid sugared cereals – because sugar only dilutes the goodness in any food. Avoid cereals which are based on refined grain or which undergo lots of re-shaping. That leaves a choice of oats, wheat germ, bran or cracked wheat – in other words, the best cereal is a do-it-yourself cereal.**

If you like muesli, make up your own out of the above (one cup of each), and keep the mixture in an airtight container in the fridge to protect it from rancidity. In the evening, take a spoonful per serving, and soak overnight in milk or fruit juice (unsweetened). This means the grains will swell before you eat them, not in your tummy. Add some dried fruit in the evening if you like. In the morning, add freshly cut fruit (any and every kind you like), and a few chopped nuts if you wish. There should be at least twice as much fruit as cereal. Home-made muesli is much, much cheaper too.

Plain oats, however, are even better food-value-for-money. If you like porridge, but don't like making it (the Kellogg survey showed that one reason working wives frequently don't cook breakfast is that they don't like coming home to washing up), use a vacuum flask. The wide-mouthed sort is a must for any nutrition-minded household. Use one ounce of rolled or whole oats for every two people if it's part of a breakfast which includes other things, one ounce per person if that's your whole breakfast. Warm the flask, put the oats in it with a good pinch of sea salt, and add a large cupful of boiling water per ounce of oats. In the morning, the porridge will be ready. Eat it with molasses or honey, not sugar – or better still, just by itself. You can 'rough up' your porridge by adding one dessertspoon of bran per person to the flask and/or the same addition of wheat germ for an extra nutritious version.

NB Most rolled oats are stabilized, just like wheat germ –

because oats are richer in oils than other cereals. It's hard to find unstabilized ones. The same comments apply to storage as to wheat germ above.

Avoiding over-processed foods has two benefits: it tends to de-concentrate your food, and at the same time, it enormously enhances your supply of the essential vitamins and minerals. The third benefit is not proved, but the 'wholeness' of foods may soon be realized as a necessary condition of their usefulness.

This is where a lot of people say 'yes in principle, but it isn't possible in modern life'. But it is. Nobody *makes* us buy tinned vegetables or frozen dinners. Foods like dessert mixes, cake mixes and ready-made pies may be handy, but they are too new for anyone to believe that they are indispensable. And getting back to making meals from basic ingredients is just a matter of habit. There is no reason why the choice of wholemeal bread, wholegrain cereals or fruit juices in a shop rather than the white flour, sugary or 'fruit drink' versions should make life any more complicated.

4. Additives – the Unknown Quantity

An additive is anything which is added to food, but which has no nutritional value itself. Like processed foods, additives are not new. Today's most used preservative, for example, sulphur dioxide, was in use 500 years ago. But just as processing now affects far more foods, and is more complicated, so are the additives used in it. About 3,000 additives are available to British manufacturers, a considerable number of which most of us wouldn't think of as additives at all – herbs, spices and vitamin C for instance.

But synthetic additive manufacture is now a thriving industry in its own right. In 1975, sales of food additives in five countries of Western Europe (including the UK) totalled over £175 million. The eight biggest selling groups are flavours, flavour enhancers (such as monosodium glutamate), thickeners and stabilizers, emulsifiers and surface active agents, food acids, colours, preservatives and antioxidants and sweeteners. The flavours market alone was worth over £70 million a year in 1975.*

Why worry about additives? The two simplest answers are: because they cause basic changes in the foods where they are used, and because many are thought to be harmful to health in their own right. Very many additives are based on natural substances, which have been known for centuries, even if they haven't always been used to do the jobs food manufacturers want them for today. They are often processed themselves to extract the exact part which the manufacturer wants. The result is an additive which is difficult to classify as natural or synthetic: it is based on something in nature, but is in a form that doesn't exist in nature. Other additives are made in laboratories, but modelled on a natural substance. The chemist makes them up to be 'nature-identical' in structure, although there is usually

* Survey by Industrial Aids, Terminal House, 52 Grosvenor Gardens, London, SW1W 0AU.

some way that they can be distinguished by analysis. Even more additives are chemical structures that don't occur in nature at all.

The common feature of additives is that they possess some property the food processor wants: they help to make food keep longer, or look more attractive, or feel different in the mouth . . . and the official way to look at additives in the UK is to classify them by such functions, into about twenty-eight groups, one of them a 'miscellaneous' category. Some groups are far larger than others: there are about 2,000 flavourings, for instance. And some are far more tightly controlled than others by law. The method of doing this is to give the food industry a 'permitted list' for a group of substances. Nothing not on the list can be used. Sometimes the maximum amount of each substance that can be used in a food is also restricted by law.

But not all groups of additives have permitted lists. In general, the tighter the control on an additive, and the shorter the permitted list for that group, the more dangerous those substances are thought to be. But some groups, such as flavourings, are restricted only by the general provision that a manufacturer must not sell anything harmful to the public. For it has been recognized for over a century that additives are potentially dangerous to the body, and need to be restricted. Very many additives have been banned when it was found they damaged health. New additives have to undergo extensive tests.

With these sort of rules, why should anyone worry about whether additives are safe? There are lots of reasons why:

1. The present Food and Drugs Act is only twenty-odd years old, and it tended to accept as safe those additives which were already established in use. But the fact that an additive has been used for a long time is no proof of its safety. I've already mentioned sulphur dioxide, and it's a good example: it is known that it is vitamin-destructive, and that sulphured food can be toxic after storage. By the way, the fact that an additive is natural is no guarantee of safety either – there are poisons in nature too. So many additives established a long time ago have never had to be safety-tested. Many have been banned on safety grounds after being used for years.
2. Even when an additive has been tested, the results mean that it is safe for the species of animals used in the tests –

not necessarily for humans.

3. Once an additive is in general use, ill-effects caused by it can be almost impossible to trace. Even a substance like thalidomide, that caused dreadful injuries, took years to be banned. An additive could even cause migraines, stomach upsets, cancer or anaemia in thousands of people, and never be traced. The most alarming example of such delayed action is cancer. Cancer can appear twenty or thirty years after contact with the cancer-inducing substance. And ill-effects can be carried on to another generation. No additive is tested for effects like these.
4. Additives mount up. Many additives are recognized as dangerous above a certain quantity. So maximum levels are set. But even if we never eat over a certain amount of any one food, no one adds up the times we eat the same additive – from different foods – in the same day. Or how much that adds up to in a year, or in five, or in ten years. Some additives are in so many common foods that several 'doses' a day are almost inevitable. Today's additive use has reached the stage where most people eat at least a dozen different ones each day. Nobody has looked at how additives interact, and what the result to health may be.
5. Additives may alter the nutritive value of food to the body.

For all these reasons, I think that the public attitude towards additives as rather a 'dirty word' is a healthy one. There are hundreds of additives which we cannot know to be safe; there is also a much smaller number which there is good reason to think dangerous at least to some of us. The short history of additive control also suggests that suspicion is the correct attitude: many additives thought to be safe have been found to be dangerous to man and banned.

The next logical question is, why are so many additives used? Why is the market for additives so healthy and fast growing? And are they really necessary ? The food industry needs additives, certainly. Some are absolutely essential to the product – they are 'built-in' to the nature of it. Some make food keep in the same condition for far longer than they would normally. Some achieve tastes, textures and colours that are not natural to the raw materials. I call these three groups built-in, convenience and cosmetic additives. Some additives do a functional *and* a cosmetic job, but generally, these two types of additives can be distinguished. In the list of additive groups later in this chapter, I'll be marking them according to their role.

Built-in Additives. Some modern food products literally couldn't exist without additives. Low-calorie soft drinks, for instance, would not be possible without saccharin. Ready-made jelly-type desserts and mousses can't be made to last and to travel without gelling agents to make and keep them solid. Others would be too dangerous without additives: a ham sandwich that sits for hours and even days in a warm pub or shop is a perfect breeding ground for bacteria. It would cause even more food poisoning cases than at present if the growth of bacteria were not retarded by preservative. From the manufacturer's viewpoint, the use of additives in foods like these is absolutely essential. But from the consumer's eye view, foods like these raise the question 'are they worth having at all?' If there is a health risk involved, why eat such foods? After all, they've only been with us a few years anyway.

Convenience additives make life easier or more profitable for the food trade – but aren't essential to the existence of the product. For instance, if you cook a steak and kidney pie at home, you wouldn't dream of adding preservative to it. So preservative isn't necessary to the food item. But in the manufacturer's view, it is to *his* steak and kidney pie. He is after the longest possible product 'life' – the name for the time a food can be stored and still remain saleable and eatable. The longer a wholesaler can store the pies, the bigger batches they can be made in, the bigger and fewer loads need be delivered to the warehouse. The longer the retailer can store the pie, the better the chances of it selling. The longer the shopper can keep it at home, the fewer complaints of foods 'going off'. So the longer the manufacturer can make his food products keep, the more popular he and his pies will be with everyone! Big scale production and deliveries, together with a good reputation for keeping, mean more profit.

Anti-mould additives in bread, anti-rancidity agents in foods containing fats, preservatives of all kinds are examples of this second type of additive. But as we've seen, they aren't strictly necessary. The food industry argues, however, that these additives do benefit the shopper – by making food cheaper to produce and distribute, and reducing wastage. They also remove much of the need for the public to pay attention to food freshness. In fact, the industry claims that 'convenience' additives keep prices down. But while some people may be prepared to run health risks for the sake of a few pennies, others might argue that it is the food trade which really benefits. Perishable foods, such as greengroceries, which do not include additives are no more expensive than additive-laden convenience foods. Though additives are becoming increasingly sophisticated, they don't seem to be bringing food prices down – or even keeping them stable. So the person who wants to put his health first doesn't have any choice.

Cosmetic additives help the manufacturer make a food product more appealing to our eyes, noses or taste buds than it would naturally be. Flavourings, the largest single group of additives used in food in this country, are dedicated to this aim. By 1900, a large proportion of those flavourings in common use were synthetic, yet even today there is still no tightly controlled 'permitted list' (although one has been proposed). This means that manufacturers can use anything they like. Colours, on the other hand, *are* tightly controlled, because so many have been found to be potential cancer-inducers.

Other cosmetic additives also alter the texture or look of food. Examples are liquid paraffin on dried fruit to make it look attractively moist – or coatings on orange skins to make them look more vivid and glossy. These sorts of additives have the least justification, yet manufacturers are determined to keep them. Their argument is clear: 'we are going to continue using them, because the British public won't buy our products without them'. The food industry has even been known to turn this statement around and say 'the public wants additives', when questioned on the need to add red colouring to blackcurrant drink for children, or on the lurid green of processed peas. Of course, the public hasn't actually been asked. Manufacturers are simply unwilling to chance their arm and offer paler peas or paler jam. They assume that housewives buy their product because they like it just as it is – colour, flavour and all.

But why do manufacturers add so many additives in dishes which the ordinary person makes equally or more successfully without additives? One answer is not encouraging for the shopper. Cosmetic additives enable manufacturers to use substitute, cheaper ingredients. Butter yellow plus a cheaper fat instead of butter; raspberry flavour instead of raspberries; emulsifiers and stabilizers instead of eggs which would normally perform that function . . . a depressing catalogue. But, say the food industrialists, why is it depressing? Provided we make something you enjoy eating, and you can't tell the difference, you, the public, are the gainer, because you are paying a lower price than the real thing would cost. Indeed, a lot of the arguments over the justification for additives boil down to cost. The food industry is convinced that the housewife wants lower costs more than she wants naturalness, flavour or even safety. Perhaps they are right, but are shoppers being given the choice? **It's only a true choice if they know what the price in health could be.**

How do you get that knowledge? If you are interested in the additives in your food, you may be tempted to buy the various regulations which control them, and which are published by Her Majesty's Stationery Office (they can also be ordered from bookshops). For this reason, I list at the end of this chapter the currently applying Statutory Instruments. But don't expect too much information from them. The regulations *are* interesting in that they give the permitted lists of additives within most groups, and often which foods are allowed to contain them. So you can find out, for instance, all the additives which, say, bread or cheese is allowed to contain. However they are written not for public understanding, but for legal control. The prose is laden with legal phraseology: 'subject to paragraph (2) of this regulation . . .', 'save as hereinafter provided', etc., and they are extremely hard to understand. The regulations make no attempt to explain what the additives are, why some are restricted and others not, etc. And the fact that an additive is allowed in, say, chocolate, doesn't mean that the producer chooses to use it. The truth is that it is extremely difficult for the public to find out either what additives are in certain food, or anything about their properties.

This is partly because the UK is still in the Dark Ages when it comes to food labels. The official attitude seems to be 'the Government will look after the safety of your food, don't you worry about it'. Until 1974, food didn't have to be labelled with any of its ingredients at all. Now additives have to be shown on foods covered by the Labelling of Food

Regulations 1970, but they don't have to be named. The manufacturer can just write 'colouring', and does not have to say whether it is natural or synthetic, or to give its name. As some groups of additives are vast (like the 2,000 flavourings, for instance), the shopper may well want to know more. Is this particular additive natural or synthetic? Is it the one which has been banned in the USA? Is it the one he recently read has been linked with skin diseases in children?

There is no way of finding out, except to write to the individual manufacturer. Although I have usually found food companies helpful, they are under no compulsion to tell a member of the public the name of the particular additive they use in a product. It is sometimes hard to understand why. Why, for instance, do Smedley list 'flavouring' on the label of HP sauce, when they could write 'clove oil'? Lots of foods do not have to be labelled with their ingredients at all. I look at what these may contain more closely later, but again, a letter to the manufacturer is the only chance of finding out what's in your favourite brand.

Three food industry arguments against labelling additives by name used to be a) that the names were too long to fit on, b) that they wouldn't mean anything to Mrs Average anyway, and c) that naming the additive would get in the way of occasional product improvements where a different flavouring etc. might be used. The last argument has some validity, but the first two don't. Additives now have numbers as well as names, so the label could say 'colour E202' for instance – not very longwinded. The second argument is the worst, because it expresses all the lack of respect that the food industry seems to have for the people who keep it in business: the shoppers. People may not understand the exact properties of polyester but they are still entitled to know that a garment is made of it and not be fobbed off with 'manmade fibre'. How much more so when their health is at stake.

Here are the families of additives you may find listed on labels, what they do and where they are used. If you know the name of the individual additive, but not which group it belongs to, try the Index. I can't include them all – there are so many chemical combinations – but I've concentrated on the ones that I think we all should be aware of.

B = built-in (essential to the existence of products)
C = convenience (isn't essential, but helps manufacturer and distributor)
Cos = cosmetic

C **Acids** give a tart flavour to food, and also adjust the alkali-acid balance. They are used in raising agents like baking powder to liberate carbon dioxide gas – which is what forces a cake to rise.

Regulated by: Miscellaneous Additives in Food Regulations 1974. No restrictions on which foods can contain them, nor on the amount to be used, except that some acids are not permitted in soft drinks or in jams or marmalade; and metatartaric acid is only permitted in wine, at 100 parts per million.

Examples: adipic, citric, fumaric, lactic, malic, phosphoric and tartaric acids. Some exist in nature, e.g. lactic acid in yoghurt, sauerkraut and soft cheese, and malic acid in fruit. They can also be products of industrial fermentation.

Typical uses: jams and marmalades (one case where use is controlled, under the Food Standards (Preserves) Order 1953); in soft drinks (controlled under Soft Drinks Regulations 1964); fruit-flavoured desserts and dessert mixes to duplicate tartness that real fruit would give; fruit-based pie fillings; sweet pickles and chutneys; one acid, metatartaric acid, is allowed only for use in wine.

Cos **Anti-caking agents** are used to prevent products from sticking together inconveniently in packets or during processing.

Regulated by: Miscellaneous Additives in Food Regulations 1974. No restrictions on what foods they can be used in nor on quantities used, except for octadecylammonium acetate, which is only permitted to be used in ammonium chloride (itself an additive) with a maximum content of 500 milligrams per kilogram.

Examples: several kinds of silicate, e.g. calcium silicate, derived from mineral sources. Calcium stearate.

Typical uses: salt, baking powder, coffee whiteners and icing sugar are commonest foods treated.

C **Anti-foaming or defoaming agents** have the property of being able to stop scum forming, or prevent liquids boiling over. Some emulsifiers also have the same function.

Regulated by: Miscellaneous Additives in Food Regulations 1974. No restrictions on the foods where they can be used, nor on how much is used, except in sugar products (under the Specified Sugar Product Regulations 1976) where anti-foaming agents in glucose syrup or dried glucose syrup (common ingredients of many processed sweet foods and confectionery) must be declared by name on the label, and the maximum level must not exceed fifteen parts per million.

Examples: oxystearin, dimethylpolysiloxane.

Typical uses: beer, wine and fruit juice processing and bottling.

C **Antioxidants** are used to prevent the deterioration that progressively affects all fats and oils when they are in contact with oxygen. Different fats break down at different rates, but the eventual result is rancidity. Most people find the flavours and smells typical of rancidity unpleasant, and it is a health problem too. The reaction between the fat and oxygen inside the body produces new substances which are irritants. They can cause disorders of the digestive tract in animals, sometimes leading to death, and retarded growth in young animals. What they do to humans has not been fully explored, although tests have started. Antioxidants grow in importance with food processing, which encourages the development of rancidity by breaking natural foods down, and then seeking to keep them edible for as long as possible.

Regulated by: Antioxidants in Food Regulations 1974. Among the tightest controlled group of additives – reflecting the recognition that they are potentially dangerous to health. The table below shows all the permitted antioxidants whose use is restricted, and what they are allowed to be used in.

Additives table

Restricted antioxidants		*Foods where they are allowed*
Propyl gallate Dodecyl gallate Octyl gallate BHA BHT	Singly or in mixtures in any of these foods	Oils Hard and soft fats Butter for manufacturing Essential oils
Ethoxyquin		Apples and pears

There are also two groups of substances with antioxidant properties that occur naturally in food. These are ascorbic acid, better known as vitamin C, and its derivatives; and tocopherols, the family to which vitamin E belongs. Both groups are used commercially as antioxidants, although the substances used are mostly synthesized 'nature-identical' versions. Vitamin C doesn't dissolve in fats, so its use is restricted to watery products: for instance, to prevent vinegar, beer, fruit juice and vegetables succumbing to the oxidation process which would darken their colour and change their flavour. Tocopherols (vitamin E is alpha tocopherol) occur naturally in oil-rich plants. Unfortunately, a large proportion is usually lost from food during processing. They are added to some foods by manufacturers. Both these groups are used freely by manufacturers, as is lecithin, a waxy substance which occurs naturally in soya beans, eggs, peanuts and some cereals, can also be synthesized, and is widely used as an emulsifer.

Synthetic antioxidants, in contrast, are tightly restricted because of persistent suspicion about their safety. Ethoxyquin is only permitted on apples and pears to delay deterioration caused by air contact during storage. Three derivatives from gallic acids are used mainly in foods which won't be subjected to much heat, which would cause them to break down. They also tend to combine with tiny traces of iron in food, producing a black discolouration. To avoid this, they are often used with a sequestering agent – another additive which will itself combine with the iron, and 'tie it up' before it can react with the gallates. Between them, the two additives may prevent the body absorbing some valuable minerals from the food.

Most controversial of the antioxidants are BHA (butylated hydroxyanisole) and BHT (butylated hydroxytoluene), which are the most effective and popular antioxidants available for animal fats. They are easy for the manufacturer to use, too, because they dissolve readily. Yet for about twenty years, they have been known to be dangerous. The UK Food Standards Committee, the Government's own additive watchdog, has twice recommended, in 1958 and again in 1963, that BHT should no longer be permitted in food. The recommendation has been ignored. The Committee based its view on an international mass of evidence which began to emerge almost as soon as these two additives went into widespread use, which was only in the early 1950s. Both BHA and BHT were found to build up in the body fat when substantial amounts are eaten. And substantial amounts *are* eaten by most people, because although the list of foods where these additives can be used looks so short, these foods are in turn ingredients in virtually every processed food there is.

BHA has been shown to produce stunted growth in young rats, and to interfere with the working of the intestinal muscles in man. BHT is even more hazardous. A variety of studies on many different animals in different countries has reported ill-effects as serious as damage to the liver and kidneys, abnormalities in offspring, poor growth in young animals, increases in blood fat and cholesterol levels and baldness. In 1972, pregnant mice given diets containing substantial amounts of BHA and BHT produced offspring suffering from abnormal behaviour and with major changes in brain chemistry. Effects reported in humans include asthma, dermatitis, tingling sensations on the skin and blistering – suggesting allergies. As a result of such evidence, BHT has been banned in many countries – yet the only reaction in Britain has been to halve the quantity of restricted antioxidants allowed in any food. The danger was acknowledged, too, by a ban on their use at all in baby and toddler food. But there are no plans either to ban BHT outright or phase it out gradually. The reason is that such a ban would cause difficulties for food processors. Antioxidants are important tools in their ever-continuing search for ways to make food keep, and sell, for ever. Synthetic antioxidants, however, are a blot on the face of food safety legislation: they prove that public safety is not always put first in food legislation.

B **Artificial sweeteners** are considered to be anything which provides sweetness without calories, excluding man-made compound sugars which don't exist in nature, but do contain calories – such as sorbitol.

Regulated by: Artificial Sweeteners in Food Regulations 1969. There are no restrictions on what foods they can be used in, nor on the maximum amount in a single food.

Example: since 1969,* only one artificial sweetener has been permitted in the UK, saccharin and two saccharin derivatives.

* 1969 was the year that sodium cyclamate was banned first in the US and then in the UK as a result of tests suggesting it was cancer-inducing in animals. Since then, it has been discovered that the tests were not reliable, and that one of the test procedures used – implanting a cyclamate pellet in the urinary bladder of mice – would have resulted in a similar number of cancers if the pellet had been a saccharin one. What's more, some of the sweeteners used did contain both cyclamate and saccharin.

Typical uses: saccharin has been used in food for almost 100 years, but the amount used has multiplied enormously in the last decade, as more and more people seek sweet foods without calories, and as manufacturers have sought an alternative to more costly sugar. Soft drinks increasingly use saccharin instead of sugar, even when they do not claim to be low in calories; low calorie cola drinks; diabetic foods.

In fact, saccharin has been under suspicion almost since it was introduced. But scattered reports of ill-effects ranging from digestive and blood clotting disorders or urticaria (itchy, swollen, patchy skin allergy) have been inconclusive so far. Still, it is banned in several European countries. In 1971, America's food standards body, the Food and Drug Administration, set maximum limits for the saccharin content of food and drinks. In 1977, saccharin finally came under threat of a complete American ban for general use following more tumours-in-test-animals studies.

C **Bases** are officially defined as 'any substance which is capable, and generally used for the purpose, of increasing the alkalinity of food'. There is more than one reason for wanting to do this: apart from altering flavour, bases may be wanted to help dissolve acidic ingredients or to react with acid in raising agents to produce carbon dioxide gas. By the way, these are the same sort of chemicals used in antacid indigestion medicines.

Regulated by: Miscellaneous Additives in Food Regulations 1974. No restrictions as to which foods may contain bases, nor on the amount to be used.

Examples: Ammonium bicarbonate, sodium carbonate, magnesium hydroxide, magnesium oxide, potassium hydroxide.

Typical uses: to control acid level of wine, tinned tomato products, olives and other foods whose acid level is too high from either a flavour or a storage point of view; in peeling solutions for potatoes, fruit, etc. in baking powder, to produce gas; in dairy products, to correct over-developed acidity. Some of these substances, such as magnesium oxide and hydroxide, are also used as indigestion remedies and laxatives. They tend to release carbon dioxide gas in the stomach, causing 'windiness' and belching; big doses may also cause kidney stones or disorders and diarrhoea; and the body tends to become dependent upon them, so that it fails to maintain its normal acid-alkali balance itself.

C **Buffers** are used to stabilize the acid-alkali balance of a food at a desired level. The object may be to maximize the keeping time of the food, to change the flavour, or to correct over-acidity. Buffers are also used to keep fizzy drinks fizzy.

Regulated by: Miscellaneous Additives in Food Regulations 1974. There's no restriction on which foods they can be used in, nor on the amount to be used.

Examples: calcium citrate, calcium diphosphate, calcium gluconate, potassium sodium tartrate, potassium malate, potassium lactate.

Typical uses: carbonated soft drinks, hundreds of processed foods including cake mixes, jams, canned potatoes, canned tomatoes and purée, baked goods.

•s/C **Bleaching agents** are officially defined as 'any substance capable of removing colour from ground bolted wheat'. In other words, they are what makes white flour really white, instead of its natural creamy colour. But most bleaching agents are also known as 'improvers', because they possess other properties which are valuable to the flour miller and baker. Bleaching agents are one of the most suspect additive groups from a health point of view. Few additives are closer to being banned in the UK.

Flour bleaches naturally if stored for several months, but storage is expensive and involves the risk of losses due to deterioration. Bleaching agents 'mature' the flour within days. At the same time, they even up the colour and baking behaviour of different wheats, in a way that millers maintain makes British wheats more acceptable and practical for large-scale baking than they would be otherwise. Other improvers also make doughs and batters easier to work with, or more consistent, for the baker.

Regulated by: Bread and Flour Regulations 1963 and Amendment 1973. The permitted agents and their uses are shown in the table below.

The bleaches and improvers suspected of being dangerous are: chlorine, chlorine dioxide (which contains chloride), potassium bromate and sulphur dioxide. Chlorine dioxide and chlorine came into use in the early 1950s to replace agene, a flour bleacher and improver banned in 1950, when it was shown to excite fits in test animals. Potassium bromate is a more recent arrival, and is now extremely widespread in bread, because it is a feature of the Chorleywood Bread Process (see p.57). None of these has satisfied either the UK

Bleaches and improvers

Where they are allowed	*Additive*	*Function*
All or any permitted in any flour except wholemeal	Benzoyl peroxide	Bleaching only, normally supplementing chlorine dioxide; 60–70 per cent of UK flour is treated with it.
	Ascorbic acid (vitamin C)	Improver only: speeds up the rearrangement of protein that takes place during the mixing and rising of yeast dough.
	Ammonium persulphate Potassium persulphate Ammonium chloride	Improvers only: they stimulate yeast development. Mainly used in some speciality breads, such as Scottish batch bread and similar breads baked in North East England.
	Monocalcium phosphate	Improver of sorts: increases acidity of dough, thus preventing development of bacteria which causes 'rope' – an infection of spores making bread smell fruity and become strand-like in texture. More common in hot weather. Also a raising agent.
	Potassium bromate	Improver only: very widely used since development of the Chorleywood Bread Process (CBP). CBP is a time-saving breadmaking method which is now used for about 75 per cent of UK bread. Potassium bromate strengthens and stabilizes the structure of dough.
	Chlorine dioxide	Bleaching and maturing agent, added by miller. Often used with other agents. About 80 per cent of UK flour for breadmaking is treated with chlorine dioxide.
	L-cysteine hydrochloride	Newest (1973) permitted improver: essential to another modern high speed breadmaking process. It accelerates the changes in protein and structure that take place naturally during breadmaking. Some of this substance occurs naturally in cereals.
Only allowed in cake flour, and not in wholemeal cake flour	Chlorine	Bleach and improver applied to about one third of UK cake flours. Acts on flour so that cakes will hold fruit better; also alleged to produce 'better eating quality and texture'.
Only allowed in biscuit flour, and not in wholemeal biscuit flour	Sulphur dioxide, also in form of sodium metabisulphite	Improvers: the first is added to flour, the second to doughs and tend to standardize the baking qualities of different wheats. About 10–15 per cent of UK biscuits contain them.

or overseas authorities that it is safe in long term use. The UK is the only EEC country that permits the use of chlorine. Potassium bromate and chlorine dioxide are currently being tested for their effects on rats by the Flour Millers and Bakers Research Association. The Association represents the baking and milling industry, and naturally wishes to show that these substances are safe enough to continue to be used. To finance these tests, a levy has been imposed on the users of the additives – a cost which of course is eventually paid by the customer. The industry has passed its first results to the Government to consider, but in its 1977 annual report, the Association said it was confident that the additives would continue to be permitted. The health hazards of sulphur dioxide are discussed under 'Preservatives'.

Colourings are the ultimate in cosmetic additives – and in many people's eyes, the least justifiable. They are not only used to intensify the existing colour of a food, but to restore the original colour lost through food processing. Two synthetic colours are added to the blackcurrant drink Ribena, for instance, because the natural deep tint of blackcurrants has been bleached by the preservative sulphur dioxide. Ribena is only an example of standard practice among manufacturers. Processed peas acquire their dramatic green hue as an apparent over-compensation by the processors for the virtually complete loss of green the peas experience through being dried, reconstituted and cooked.

Besides masking processing, colourings can be used to make a food look as if it contains more of a certain ingredient than it does. They make possible such economies as black cherry yoghurt with few cherries, but plenty of cherry colour. And as I have said, the ingredient may even be entirely absent. This is the case whenever a food carries the word 'flavour' in the name on the label. That means that the item preceding it – be it vanilla, butter, strawberry or cheese – isn't there at all! It is, as it were, merely represented by the appropriate colouring and flavouring additives. Colours can be produced to copy the tint of any natural food.

Not surprisingly, the use of colours in food is increasing fast, as a way of cutting down the cost of raw materials. Manufacturers defend colourings as something that makes food more attractive – as if they are doing the public a favour. They also maintain that shoppers insist on certain items having a certain colour, and that they will not buy the goods without it. Indeed, Marks and Spencer have tried offering undyed peas and other foods alongside the coloured ones. They did not sell. But does this prove anything? If all peas were pale, as in France, they clearly would sell.

Regulated by: Colouring Matter in Food Regulations 1973. Only eighteen synthetic dyes, plus nineteen colours obtained from natural materials, are permitted in UK food. The reason for the tight control is that so many colours have in the past been found to be cancer-inducing in test animals – even after years of being eaten by the unsuspecting public. But the banning of dye after dye isn't reassuring: it simply suggests that synthetic dyes, which are derived from coal tar, are basically extremely dangerous. It is virtually impossible to trace cancer to its cause, which may have been met many years before. Of the thirty dyes on the first permitted list of colours from 1957, fewer than half are still allowed. Seven new ones have been introduced, but more are under suspicion. Only four of the eighteen dyes on the present UK list are also permitted as safe both by the EEC and the US. In 1973, EEC influence resulted in seven UK colours not considered safe being discontinued, and replaced by six new ones, plus three for limited use only.

But new dangers are still being realized. For example, in 1971 a red dye, Ponceau MX, was banned as a result of safety (or rather danger) tests carried out by the British Industrial Biological Research Association (known as BIBRA, and the main non-industry test body for additives in the UK). On 1 January 1976, Orange RN – a tint widely used in soft drinks, readymade desserts, sweets, soup mixes, meat and fish spreads and also cosmetics – was banned following tests showing that it damaged the red blood corpuscles and livers of pigs in a permanent manner. Amaranth, one of the red colourings that used to be thought safe in the EEC, US and UK, was banned in 1976 in the US (where it is called Red Dye 2). As long ago as the late 1960s, Russian additive testers had published studies showing that Amaranth caused birth defects, stillbirths and cancer in laboratory animals. The American Food and Drug Administration eventually carried out tests of its own, and confirmed that chick embryos exposed to Amaranth suffered deformities such as incomplete skeletons and stunted growth. There are no plans to ban Amaranth in the UK, where it is equally widely used. Three more dyes were banned from food as from 1 January 1977 because of EEC pressure to produce a list of colourings acceptable by common European safety standards.

The list below shows all the present permitted synthetic dyes, although I cannot help thinking that between writing this and publication day, the list will almost certainly be rendered out of date by some new danger discovery.

UK permitted food dyes as of March 1977

† Amaranth
† Black PN
† Brilliant blue FCF
† Brown FK
† Carmoisine
Chocolate brown FB
† Chocolate brown HT
Erythrosine BS
† Green S
Indigo carmine
Orange G
† Patent blue V
† Ponceau 4R
Quinoline yellow
Red 2G
Sunset yellow FCF
Tartrazine
† Yellow 2G

The ten dyes marked with daggers are considered unsafe by international standards. The EEC has set a deadline: if more satisfactory proof of their safety cannot be produced by the end of 1978, they will all be banned.

You may be curious about which colours are in which foods you eat: unfortunately, telling you what tint each produces would be no great guide. Green S, for instance, is basically a green colour, but is used in red foods too. Orange tints can be used with other dyes to produce a variety of colour effects. (See my comments on labelling earlier in this chapter.) Brown FK is used in many foods, but notably in kippers (FK stands for For Kippers), where it and smoke flavour enable the processor to bypass the traditional smoking technique which would brown the kipper naturally. Brown FK is a good instance of how the food industry feels about colour additives. Although it was shown almost ten years ago that Brown FK in large doses damaged the heart and muscles of rats, guinea pigs and mice, the food industry feels its use is justified – even though in 1975 more tests showed that half of one milligram of Brown FK (you'd easily eat that much in one kipper) could set off cancer-like changes in samples of cells, under laboratory conditions. But, say the kipper makers, we must go on using it because without it, the housewife won't buy kippers. They don't seem to have realized that dye-less kippers – Manx ones – are already bought; or that if *all* kippers were pale, this would become the standard, and people would find them ordinary.

So certain is the food industry of its absolute need for colourings to add to foods – and to replace some food ingredients – that thirteen different branches of the industry have joined together to finance an effort to produce safety evidence. They include the trade associations of makers of soft drinks, sweets, chocolate, cider, ice cream, meat and bacon, cakes and biscuits, sauces and pickles, canned fruit and vegetables, jam, soup, gravy and even glacé cherries! They are concentrating on six of the suspect dyes: Amaranth, Carmoisine, Brilliant blue FCF, Chocolate Brown HT, Green S and Ponceau 4R. But how can any additives with such poor safety records be justified? Especially when they are added to foods only for cosmetic reasons, or to cover up substitute or inferior ingredients? Food colours are intended to persuade shoppers that something is better quality than it really is.

B or C **Diluents** are substances in which additives can be dissolved or with which they can be diluted, in order to put them into a form which can be added to food.

Regulated by: usually regulations for the particular additive they are used to carry, i.e. colouring diluents are described under the Colour in Food regulations. But any substance not specifically banned for use in food may be used as a diluent for bread additives.

Example: acetic acid, an acid naturally present in vinegar, but also produced as a laboratory product, is used to dissolve colouring additives.

B **Edible gums** are derived from plants and used to thicken very many manufactured products, giving them a desired texture and in some cases, stability of consistency during transport and handling.

Regulated by: Emulsifiers and Stabilisers in Foods Regulations 1975.

Examples: acacia, carob, ghatti, guar, karaya, tragacanth. Used in foods such as ready-made desserts, mousses, chutney and pickles, custards, cheesecakes, pie fillings. Not additives that need to be worried about.

B or C **Emulsifiers and stabilizers** are usually considered together, because the substances in these classes often perform both functions. Emulsifiers are substances which have the property of enabling oil and water to mix – or oily and watery ingredients. Stabilizers help keep such combinations from separating, also preserving the texture of foods which would be spoiled by joggling. There are natural and synthetic substances in both classes.

Regulated by: Emulsifiers and Stabilisers in Foods Regulation 1975.

Examples (table below). Emulsifiers and stabilizers have attracted less suspicion than some other food additives, but some from these widely used groups have unsatisfactory safety reputations. While lecithin, for example, is a positive asset to a food in the same way as added vitamins would be, sodium carboxymethylecellulose, one of the cellulose derivatives, has been reported to cause tumours in rats. But the results of studies in both the USA and Canada, in 1969 and 1961 respectively, have not been officially accepted. Polyoxyethylene compounds have been in use as anti-staling agents in baked goods for about 30 years. Ten years after their introduction, tests had already suggested that animals fed substantial amounts of these compounds developed liver and intestinal damage rapidly. There was a proposal that the additives should be banned, but the food industry managed to avert this. While GMS (see table) and similar fats could be described as 'natural', they have been altered so far from the way they occur in nature that they are really synthetic, with the extra anxiety about safety that this implies.

Emulsifying salts are mixtures of mineral salts which make the mixing of certain foods possible, and keep the result stable.

Regulated by: Emulsifiers and Stabilisers in Foods Regulations 1975.

Examples: usually given on labels as 'emulsifying salts', because the blend used is often complex. Main use in processed cheeses and cheese spreads.

Excipients are 'carriers' for dry ingredient additives, to put them into a convenient form.

Regulated by: no specific regulations. Any non-prohibited substance can be used.

Examples: lactose, the chemical name for milk sugar, is used as an excipient to make up vitamins into vitamin tablets; some excipients are used to carry the improvers and bleaches in bread.

Firming agents make vegetables and fruit crisper and crunchier, so that they don't seem processed.

Regulated by: Miscellaneous Additives Regulations 1974.

Emulsifiers and stabilizers

Example	*Group*	*Sources*	*Typically used to:*
Agar agar Carrageen Sodium alginate	Members of large group of seaweed extracts	Various seaweeds	Jell and stabilize desserts, mixes, chutneys, baked goods, ice cream, processed meals, salad dressings, spreads.
Lecithin	Fatty compound containing phosphorus and vitamins inositol and choline. Present in all body cells and made by body	Soya beans	Soften crumb in bread and cakes, emulsify margarine, stabilize chocolate.
Pectin	Family name for group of substances	Apples, sugar beet, citrus fruit	Set preserves, solidify confectionery, stabilize pickle or desserts.
Glyceryl monostearate (GMS)	Most familiar of large sophisticated group of fats known as super-glycerinated i.e. combined with glycerol. Also known as fatty esters of glycerol	Animal, vegetable or synthetic	Boost rising power of bread, cakes, and soften crumb; affect texture and aid cutting in confectionery; help mixing in ice cream, dessert mixes, soup etc.; delay staling.
Methyl cellulose	One of several cellulose derivatives, not digestible by body, but able to swell up many times by absorbing fluid, and then form a stable mass	Cotton, wood or synthetic	Add body to 'slimming' foods, pie fillings, meringues, ice cream and lollies.
Sorbitan or **Polyoxyethylene stearate**	Members of sophisticated group made by combining the sugar/alcohol sorbitol with fatty acids for sorbitans, more recently adding ethylene oxides as well for poly-group	Synthesized	Hold moisture, disperse fat in sweets, chocolate; release flavour quickly; improve texture in confectionery, ice cream.
Sodium phosphate	See *Emulsifying salts*		

No limit is set to their use, except for aluminium potassium sulphate, which is not accepted except for use on glacé cherries, where the maximum level is restricted.

Examples: the commonest agents are calcium salts, which are added to blanched vegetables intended for freezing or canning to restore crispness, or to pickles to give more 'crunch'. Sugar and Epsom salts also act as firming agents.

Cos

Flavourings are the largest single group of food additives, and also the group whose use is thought to be growing fastest. About 2,000 substances are in use in EEC countries. They not only enable manufacturers to season foods, as one would at home, but to give the impression that an ingredient has been used when it hasn't. This, say manufacturers, keeps ingredient costs down and therefore benefits the housewife. Other reasons for using flavour additives are to even out the differences in taste which naturally exist between different batches of ingredients – producing a 'consistent' product – another claimed benefit to the consumer; and to restore flavour lost by processing.

Regulated by: there are no 'permitted lists' of natural or synthetic flavourings, so manufacturers are free to use any substance subject to the general provision that they should not add anything which would be harmful. This loose control is to be tightened, following a Report in 1976 suggesting that such a free use of flavourings was not desirable, given the large number of untested and synthetic substances in use.

Examples: heat acetic acid with ethyl alcohol and you get a flavour which will give a peachy, pear-like or apple-ish taste to foods. As the enormous number of flavouring additives suggests, almost any food manufacturer can find one to use in his product. Although many are natural herbs, spices and flavourings such as vanilla, many others are laboratory-constructed compounds. Butter flavour, cheese flavour, fruit flavours and smoke flavours are a few widely used varieties, which may include mixtures of natural extracts and synthetic compounds.

The biggest question mark against flavourings is the fact that few have been safety-tested unless they are recent introductions.

/B

Gelling agents are substances which can turn liquids into jellies, see under *Emulsifiers and Stabilizers*, above.

Cos **Glazing agents** give the outside of food a protective and/or decorative glossy finish.

Regulated by: Miscellaneous Additives Regulations 1974. There are no restrictions on the foods which can be glazed, nor on levels of use, except for carnauba wax. This hard wax obtained from the Brazilian wax palm is used to polish confectionery, and this is its only permitted use. Level of use is restricted to 200 milligrams per kilogram of food.

Examples: chocolate confectionery may be given an attractive sheen by glazing, and also a crisp-edged looking shape, by using a waxy fat such as sorbitan monostearate; shellac, an insect-derived resin, paraffin wax, beeswax, dextrin and various synthesized fats are other glazing agents used for such foods as sweets, chewing gum, cheese rings.

Dried fruit is glazed with mineral oil, also known as liquid paraffin, which keeps it looking appealingly glossy and 'fresh' for months. It also aids mechanical packing, by preventing the stickiness of the fruit gumming up machines.

Mineral oils are only permitted on a small number of foods, apart from dried fruit, because they are not accepted as safe. The oil inhibits the body from absorbing fat-soluble vitamins during digestion. In addition, oil can accumulate within the body. With prolonged use, mineral oil has been known to be carried in droplets to lymph nodes in the body, causing lumps. Lipoid pneumonia has been reported following the use of mineral oil in nasal drops or sprays – not very different from eating it. Washing dried fruit in hot water removes some of the mineral oil from it. In 1976, a Government-requested Report recommended that alternatives be sought for mineral oil, and that the amount used on dried fruit be reduced.

C **Humectants** improve the storage life of foods by preventing them from becoming dried out by the natural evaporation of water. The substances used are chosen for their moisture-retaining properties.

Regulated by: Miscellaneous Additives Regulations 1974. There are no restrictions as to which foods humectants may be used in, nor on the levels of use.

Examples: sorbitol, a sugar which is a man-made arrangement of natural sugars, is used as a humectant in sweets, shredded coconut, jelly-type confectionery, marshmallows, some ice cream and chocolates. Glycerol or glycerine, and mannitol are other humectants related to sorbitol.

B **Liquid freezants** are substances which extract heat from food, so that bringing food into contact with them freezes it. They are liquids or liquefied gases.

Regulated by: Miscellaneous Additives in Foods Regulations 1974. Can be used in any foods to any amount.

Examples: nitrogen gas, used in foods that need to be frozen quickly, e.g. strawberries. It also acts as a *Packaging gas*, below.

B **Packaging gas** is a gas which is forced into an empty package in order to displace the oxygen already there. The package is then filled with food, which is protected from the destructive effects of oxygen contact, i.e. oxidation, where oxygen causes food structure to change, leading to off-flavours and rancidity.

Regulated by: Miscellaneous Additives Regulations 1974. The gases may be used in any food, to any amount.

Examples: foods containing oils are the main ones vulnerable to oxidation, and are often packed using nitrogen gas. Examples are nuts and coffee.

/C/ os **Preservatives** slow down or stop the natural deterioration of food caused when yeast, bacteria or mould feed on it. The official description is 'any substance which is capable of inhibiting, retarding or arresting the growth of micro-organisms or any deterioration of food due to micro-organisms *or of masking the evidence of any such deterioration*', an extra function which is not appealing.

It must be agreed that preservatives do have more justification for their use than merely cosmetic additives. Food spoilage not only causes waste, and prevents regular supplies out of season, but some of the micro-organisms produced are harmful or dangerous to man. Examples are the salmonella organisms most often associated with food poisoning, and botulins, fungi-like organisms which are fatal to man in even minute quantities. Many meat products would be too dangerous to eat after storage if preservatives were not used.

However, the fact that preservatives can protect us should not blind us to the risk they themselves carry. Many people feel that preservatives are used unnecessarily often, almost as a 'put it in for luck' policy, in foods where they aren't needed, if proper hygiene and care are exercised in handling and processing. And, as I have already said, the use of preservatives to enable foods to be kept on sale for enormously long periods of time is not to protect the eater, but to increase the profitability of the product. It does this by reducing losses in storage, making possible bulk manufacture and long storage, and giving the shopper confidence in the 'everlasting' quality of the food.

Regulated by: Preservatives in Food Regulations 1975, which gives a list of the permitted substances. Substances which are ordinary food ingredients but also have a preserving action are not restricted and these include vinegar, sugar, salt, herbs, spices, curing and smoking, spirits, wines and hop extract.

Examples: the most widely used preservative in Britain is almost certainly sulphur dioxide, a colourless gas which has multiple attractions for food processors. It preserves the flavour and appearance of food, particularly the colour, which is kept light when it would naturally darken. It is therefore popular with manufacturers of such varied products as fruit juice (preserving colour and flavour), sultanas (keeping them pale); sausages and sausage meat (killing bacterial growth and retaining colour of 'fresh' meat); flour for biscuits (improving baking performance and keeping flour white); and wine and beer (preserving pale colour).

We all eat some sulphur dioxide every single day, and most of us more than once a day, as the table of uses (p.97) shows.

The growth in the use of sulphur dioxide is illustrated by a use which wouldn't have been thought of even 15 years ago – in pre-prepared potatoes. Today few restaurants prepare their own potatoes, especially for chips. They are delivered, pre-peeled and chopped, in large polythene bags where they sit in a sulphur dioxide-impregnated environment. This preserves their pale colour. It also preserves the vitamin C content. But a great deal is still unknown about the chemical nature of sulphur dioxide. For instance, much of the sulphur dioxide in food disappears or at least cannot be detected after a period of storage. In a sealed food, it must have gone somewhere. What does it turn into? Sulphur dioxide is known to be a reactive chemical, which can easily interact with others.

Although sulphur dioxide helps preserve vitamin C in foods, it destroys vitamin B1, thiamin. It would be quite easy for someone living mainly on processed foods, and drinking beer, cider or wine regularly, to lose most of their vitamin B1 supply in this way. The result would be a deficient nervous system, quickly causing digestive upsets,

Sulphur dioxide – permitted uses

Food	*Maximum amount Milligrams per kilogram*
Beer	70
Candied peel	100
Cider	200
Flour for biscuits	200
Fruit, canned	350
Fruit, crystallized	100
Fruit, dried	2,000
Fruit juices	800
Hamburgers	450
Jam	100
Perry	200
Pickles and sauces	100
Potatoes – raw, peeled	50
Potatoes, dried	550
Sausages	450
Sausage meat	450
Soft drinks	350
Sugar	70
Tomato pulp/purée	350
Vegetables, dried	2,000
Vinegar	70
Wine	450

irritability or depression. A second health worry is that some foods treated with sulphur dioxide have been found to be toxic after storage. This is serious when long storage is just what sulphur dioxide is used to achieve.

But a more recent suspicion is the most worrying of all. Sulphur dioxide is suspected of encouraging genetic mutations – changes in characteristics passed on to offspring – because it has an active effect on nucleic acids, the proteins which are the basic building blocks of life, and which carry on our characteristics to the next generation. The body can dispose of sulphur dioxide as it can many other unwanted substances, but nobody knows exactly how much we can handle. The legal limits on the amount which can be used do not take into account the many different foods we may eat with sulphur dioxide in a single day.

In 1959, the Food Standards Committee Report on Preservatives expressed reservations about the widening use of sulphur dioxide, particularly on potatoes, or where it might be used for the purposes of deceiving people into thinking meat was fresh when it wasn't. Both these are cosmetic or convenience, not safety, uses. At that time, they calculated that the average person ate about 15 to 20 milligrams of sulphur dioxide per day. But in the 1970s, that estimate is ludicrously low. It is almost certain to be exceeded by anyone who regularly drinks wine or beer, or who often eats in catering establishments.

Eating out is a particularly sulphur-dioxide-rich situation, because foods sold in catering establishments are allowed to contain ten per cent more of the additive than foods sold for home consumption. **A combination of eating school meals and drinking soft drinks means that many children eat a lot of sulphur dioxide. Children are far more vulnerable to ill-effects from additives, both because they have a lower body weight – so the additive is in a relatively larger quantity – and because the body's enzyme systems for disposing of unwanted substances may not be well-developed yet.**

Nitrates and nitrites are two other groups of preservatives widely used, and thoroughly suspect on safety grounds. They are mainly functional, used to prevent potentially dangerous bacterial and fungal growth in animal foods, particularly delicatessen-type cooked meats and sausages, and canned meat products. Salamis, pâtés, liver sausage, corned beef . . . they are almost always preserved with sodium or potassium nitrate or nitrite. But these additives have another attraction for meat processors. They are what gives pickled and cured meat its distinctive pink colour. Have you ever wondered why bacon is such a different colour from pork? Nitrates can occur naturally in many foods, both vegetables and meat, and they have been used for centuries to cure meat as saltpetre. Unfortunately, this does not mean that they are safe.

The doubts arise because our digestive systems, under certain conditions, can turn nitrates into nitrites. The nitrites then affect the blood in such a way that it cannot carry the proper amount of oxygen around the body. In small quantities, the body can 'disarm' the nitrites, but large amounts of nitrites can literally suffocate us. There are several cases a year of this happening to small infants, who have been seriously ill or died following an accidentally big intake of nitrate. The most likely way for this to happen is when nitrates become concentrated in water, which is then used to make up baby feeds. Such nitrate concentration happens easily in summer, when natural nitrate levels are highest, but also when farmers are using nitrate fertilizers which then dissolve in rain and accumulate in rivers which feed reservoirs. As the use of fertilizers has risen, so has this risk. But although infants are most at risk, anyone can be affected by high nitrate levels.

Another hazard of nitrates and nitrites which has recently been under debate is whether they may encourage cancer. Though the mechanism is far from clear, it seems that the body may under some circumstances turn the nitrates or nitrites in processed meat into substances called nitrosamines during digestion. Many nitrosamines are proven cancer-encouragers. The risk came to light following an outbreak of liver cancer among cattle in Norway. The disease was traced to the fish meal the cattle were being fed on – and which had been treated with nitrates. The theory is controversial because of the fact that nitrates occur naturally – suggesting that any cancer-causing effect would have been noticed long ago. But we don't know whether there may be a different reaction in the body to extra, added nitrates; or what difference added amounts may make. Some people at least may not be able to cope with more than a certain amount of nitrates – and as cancer may not develop until years after exposure to its cause, any relationship is very hard to prove.

So why are nitrates and nitrites still permitted? The short and discouraging answer is because they are irreplaceable as yet in the eyes of the food industry. No alternative substance is known which would do their useful job. People won't buy ham and bacon unless it is pink, say the pork processors. And delicatessen counters and corned beef couldn't exist – they'd be too dangerous – without the nitrate and nitrite families. Both the Food Standards Committee and food manufacturers would be relieved if a safer alternative could be found – but until it is, it's a risk that they consider we must take. As more of us rely on pre-cooked meals and delicatessen counters, it is a risk we are taking more often. Nitrates and nitrites are permitted in pickled meat at 200 parts per million in cooked meat, and 500 parts per million in uncooked meat.

The different rates are to take account of the effect of cooking, which tends to reduce the nitrite content in food. But the amount of reduction varies widely, even when the same method of cooking is used. When the Food Standards Committee tested 95 samples of cooked meat, some fried, some boiled, some grilled, for their 1959 Preservatives Report, they found that some samples lost 90 per cent of their nitrites, but others only 20 per cent, even when cooked the same way. Frying seemed most nitrite-destructive – but frying has other disadvantages.

Unfortunately, delicatessen meats get no further cooking at all. And more unfortunately, the amount of nitrate in food increases when the meat is stored. In uncooked meat, it doesn't increase fast, and the meat would probably be obviously 'off' before the nitrite level had risen alarmingly high. But when meat is cooked, the level increases fast, especially in sliced or minced meat. So pre-packed, sliced bacon, sausage, salami and ham can have very high amounts if they have been stored in a shop or in the home for a few days.

The only other foods where nitrites and nitrates are permitted in Britain are cheeses – any cheese except for Cheddar and Cheshire-type hard cheeses and soft cheeses. The Dutch Government also allows nitrate in Edam and Gouda; France does not. Some cheesemaking methods, such as are used for hard cheeses, naturally produce a preserving substance, nisin. So these are cheeses which do not easily go bad. The cheeses where manufacturers like to add preservative are the low acid, somewhat sweet varieties such as Dutch, Samsoe, Emmenthal, etc. Up to 1962, no preservatives were allowed in cheese sold in Britain. Now you can't tell where they have been used and where not, because cheese does not have to show its ingredients under the Food Labelling Regulations.

Another flavour-preserving additive is benzoic acid, a white crystalline powder. By law, it can be used in Britain in coffee and tea liquid extracts, in colouring additives, in flavouring additives, in crystallized fruit, in processed fruit and tomatoes, in pickles, in fruit juices, in soft drinks and in fruit yoghurt. The restriction on its use reflects some doubt about its safety: although benzoic acid occurs in nature (mainly in berries), when it has been given to test rats and mice, young rodents suffered retarded growth, nerve disorders and a lower survival rate.

Calcium propionate is often used in bread and other baked goods, particularly in hotter weather, to discourage the development of fungal and mould organisms, particularly 'rope' which would shorten the sales life of the bread. The use of preservative thus prolongs the appearance of freshness.

Apples and oranges may be packed in wrappers impregnated with diphenyl to prevent deterioration from mould or fungus; sorbic acid and related substances prevent deterioration in cheese, chocolates and cakes.

B **Propellents** are gases or active liquids which help propel foods from aerosol containers.

Regulated by: Miscellaneous Additives Regulations 1974. No restrictions are placed on which foods they can be used with, nor on amounts used.

Examples: the UK has few examples of aerosol-packed foods so far, but nitrous oxide is the propellent used for aerosol-packed 'cream' toppings.

C **Release agents** prevent food from sticking to containers, trays or moulds. They are usually oil or wax derivatives.

Regulated by: Miscellaneous Additives Regulations 1974. They may be used with any food, and to whatever level the manufacturer wishes, with a few exceptions.

Examples: sophisticated fats called polyglycerol esters of fatty acids of soya bean oil are used to grease baking tins – their only permitted use. Beeswax is sometimes used to prevent confectionery sticking together.

3/Cos **Sequestrants** prevent deterioration in food which would be caused by the presence of minerals which encourage oxidation; e.g. an iron-rich food literally rusts as the oxygen reacts with the iron. The sequestrant combines with the mineral, inactivating it and sometimes preventing other unwanted effects, e.g. too-quick setting in dessert mixes, caused by concentration of calcium.

Regulated by: Miscellaneous Additives Regulations 1974.

Examples: calcium disodium stops mineral reactions which would darken fruit drinks, tinned fruit and vegetables and pre-made salads. Although sequestrants help preserve vitamin C, by preventing oxygen action, they may also render minerals in food unavailable to humans, for whom they are vital nutrients. The increasing use of soft drinks and processed produce means that the use of sequestrants is rising; and therefore the amount of minerals available from the produce may be falling.

C **Solvents** are liquids in which additives are 'carried' in order to make it possible to incorporate them into foods. Solvents are also used to extract elements from food, in which case they are themselves usually undesirable food ingredients, intended to be removed before processing is completed.

Regulated by: Permitted Solvents Regulations 1967. There is a permitted list of solvents, but they can be used in any foods, and to any amount. So far, the regulations do not restrict the amount of solvent residue which can remain in food when a solvent is used to extract elements from ingredients.

Examples: apart from water, the most common solvents used for extraction are based on alcohol, for resins, and on ether, for fats. Ethyl acetate is used to dilute colour additives, among other solvents. Trichlorethylene was used in America to extract caffeine from coffee beans to make decaffeinated coffee. The question of solvent residues hit the headlines two years ago, when the trichlorethylene remaining in the decaffeinated coffee was accused of being dangerous to health (a different extraction method is used in Europe, by the way).

C **Stabilizers** – see *Emulsifiers and Stabilizers*.

Action

If you've found this chapter depressing, I can't blame you. The situation on a national scale is not encouraging: the use of additives is going to go on increasing, with the rise in convenience foods, and the decline of small companies. Larger companies seek large-scale production, greater economy of ingredients and longer storage life for their products. They are often more scrupulous about hygiene, and ingredient standards, than smaller producers, but the size of their operations makes preserving additives more attractive.

But the situation for you, personally, need not be depressing at all. Think the other way round: of all the foods which contain no additives at all, and of the many more where the additives are ones which are harmless – natural flavourings, gelling agents, lecithin – for instance.

Avoiding processed foods automatically frees you from having to bother at all about the vast majority of additives: there are none at all in so many basic foods.

No-additive foods

Fresh fruit (peeled or scrubbed)	Fresh meat
Fresh milk	Vegetables

Eggs	Vegetable oils
Fresh fish	Wholemeal flour
Dried beans and peas	Rice, oats, barley, etc.
Hard cheese (except vegetable colouring)	Yoghurt (natural)
Honey, treacle, molasses, raw sugar	Nuts, peanuts, coconut
Coffee, tea, fruit juices	Dried figs and dates

Then there are all the foods which exist in 'with additive' and 'without additive' versions:

★ Wholemeal bread (from conscientious health food shop or home-made)

★ Cottage cheese (read the label to check for preservative)

★ Yoghurt with fruit (must show preservative on the label if used)

★ Dried raisins (Sun-Maid are additive-free; some are packed with vegetable oil instead of mineral oil; or from health food store)

★ Other dried fruit (pale dried fruit is usually treated with sulphur dioxide – apricots, apple slices, sultanas. But some health food shops sell unsulphured versions)

Which to avoid

However, there will also be foods which you would like to use which do contain additives. And it is not realistic to say 'I'm never going to eat anything containing an additive again'. The answer is a compromise, where one tries to choose the brands with the fewest additives, and makes a special effort to avoid the additives most suspected of being undesirable. Which are these?

Colourings are probably one of the most 'worth avoiding' groups. They serve no useful purpose, and have a poor safety record. But some colourings are harmless: anatto (used in butter and red cheeses), the spice turmeric (which adds the yellow colour to curry powder), carotene (vegetable colouring similar to what's present in carrots), beetroot-derived red, and cochineal (made from an insect) are examples of colourings which are acceptable to most of us. So isn't it a pity that food labels rarely state which colour has been used? This is an example of where it is worth writing to the food manufacturer, and asking what the colouring he uses in product 'x' is. They are usually helpful and informative.

Nitrates and nitrites in delicatessen meats and pies are a second suspect group: especially in pre-sliced meats, where the nitrate level rises fast, and there's no cooking either, to reduce it again. Nitrates and nitrites are usually declared by name on labels, or as 'preservatives' on tags near the food on delicatessen counters. But there are meats which don't contain them. Watch out for them.

Antioxidants are worth avoiding – but it's hard to do so, without eliminating *all* foods containing processed fats from your shopping list. It can be done – it just means avoiding shop-made cakes, biscuits, lard, ice cream, pies, pastry, etc. Make them from scratch, and there's no problem.

Sulphur dioxide is another additive which is hard to avoid – and impossible, if you want to go on drinking beer and wine. In this case, the best course is probably to resign yourself, and simply cut down on the amount you take in from processed foods. Except for dried fruit sulphur dioxide is almost never named on labels, but the family function'preservative' is used.

Additives aren't something that need turn you into a worried hypochondriac, but they are an extra, and often unnecessary, risk in life. If you want to know where they are, letters to the manufacturers of foods are almost always courteously answered. If you'd like tighter controls on the use of additives, write and tell your MP so. You may also like to write to an MP who has made food safety her special interest: Mrs Joyce Butler, c/o the House of Commons.

As heartening thoughts to end a worrying chapter, I'd like to remind you of all the foods you can eat and enjoy that are additive-free; of the fact that less than a hundred years ago, we did without most additive-laden foods without noticeable hardship; and that if you eat a meal in a really top class restaurant, your food is likely to be additive-free, because they'll be cooking from basic materials. If they can, why can't you?

I finished this chapter after a short visit to a Greek island. For the time I was there, I don't think I ate any additives at all – yet I can't remember nicer food.

STATUTORY INSTRUMENTS CONCERNED WITH ADDITIVES IN UK FOOD

There are three kinds of additive regulations. One controls what goes into a single category of food – into cheese, or cream, for instance. The other controls a category of additives – preservatives or colouring, for instance. The two kinds need to be read together to make sense. Otherwise, the Cheese Regulations may madden you by referring to a paragraph in the Preservative in Food Regulations, for instance. The third type covers unintentional additives – i.e. contaminants like lead.

Year	*No.*	*Title*
1951	1196	Food Standards (Edible Gelatine) Order 1951
	2240	Food Standards (Edible Gelatine) Commencement Order 1951
1953	691	Food Standards (Preserves) Order 1953
1959	831	Arsenic in Food Regulations 1959
	2106	Fluorine in Food Regulations 1959
1961	1931	Lead in Food Regulations 1961
1962	721	Milk and Dairies (Emulsifiers and Stabilizers) Regulations 1962
	1531	Milk and Dairies (Preservatives) Regulations 1962
1963	1435	Bread and Flour Regulations 1963
1964	19	Meat Treatment Regulations 1964
	760	Soft Drinks Regulations 1964
1966	1073	Mineral Hydrocarbons in Food Regulations 1966
	1074	Butter Regulations 1966
1967	1582	Solvents in Food Regulations 1967
	1866	Ice-Cream Regulations 1967
	1867	Margarine Regulations 1967
	1939	Solvents in Food (Amendment) Regulations 1967
1969	1817	Artificial Sweeteners in Food Regulations 1969
	1818	Soft Drinks (Amendment) Regulations 1969
1970	94	Cheese Regulations 1970
	400	Labelling of Food Regulations 1970
	752	Cream Regulations 1970
1972	1117	Milk (Special Designation) (Amendment) Regulations 1972
	1391	Bread and Flour (Amendment) Regulations 1972

	1510	Labelling of Food (Amendment) Regulations 1972
	1939	Poisons Rules 1972
1973	1052	Arsenic in Food (Amendment) Regulations 1973
	1053	Lead in Food (Amendment) Regulations 1973
	1340	Colouring Matter in Food Regulations 1973
1974	1120	Antioxidants in Food Regulations 1974
	1121	Miscellaneous Additives in Food Regulations 1974
	1122	Cheese (Amendment) Regulations 1974
1975	1484	Fluorine in Food (Amendment) Regulations 1975
	1485	Miscellaneous Additives in Food (Amendment) Regulations 1975
	1486	Emulsifiers and Stabilizers in Food Regulations 1975
	1487	Preservatives in Food Regulations 1975
1976	103	Skimmed Milk with Non-Milk Fat (Amendment) Regulations 1976
	509	Specified Sugar Products Regulations 1976
	541	Cocoa and Chocolate Product Regulations 1976

5. To Eat Meat, or Not to Eat Meat?

One big stumbling block for would-be converts to healthy eating seems to be their notion that it would mean giving up meat. The association in most people's minds between 'healthy eating' and vegetarianism is strong, and anyone who works in the health food business finds themselves constantly asked if they are vegetarian. **But is it necessary to be vegetarian to eat healthily? The answer is no, but there are good reasons for most people to eat *less* meat.**

Vegetarians are correct in saying that you do not need to eat meat or fish to be well nourished. It is more difficult to have a well-balanced diet if you also eliminate dairy produce – cheese, milk, yoghurt – as vegans do. Some vegetarians will eat eggs, others won't. Vegans never do.

Meat and fish are good sources of protein, fat, iron, vitamins A and D, and the B vitamins. But all these elements can be obtained by eating other foods – particularly dairy foods. Although meat is a concentrated source of protein, this is no great advantage. What you want is a reasonable quantity of protein *per calorie*. The chart below shows how other foods can be just as good protein sources.

There used to be a theory among nutritionists that there were 'First Class' proteins and 'Second Class' ones, based on which foods contained all the essential amino acids, the different substances in the protein family. 'Essential' was used to mean the amino acids the body has to obtain from outside – opinions vary as to whether there are eight or ten of these which the body cannot manufacture itself. Meat and fish and dairy foods contain all of them, so they were considered 'First Class'. Everything else was 'Second Class'.

But now most nutritionists think this distinction is wrong – for two reasons. First, they have realized that people do not usually eat one particular food in isolation. So the different proteins in different foods eaten together – bread and peanut butter, beans on toast – can add up to a meal which provides all the different amino acids. Secondly, the pattern of meat protein – the relative amounts of the different amino acids – used to be thought of as the ideal, a standard by which all other foods should be judged. That idea is now seen as arbitrary. For the truth is, nobody really knows exactly how much of which amino acids we do need. There are so many examples of perfectly healthy individuals in this country who have eaten little or no meat or fish in their whole lives, that it is clear that these particular protein combinations are not essential.

Protein in food – meat isn't everything

Men need about 60–70 grams a day; women need 50–60.

Example of food	*Protein grams per ounce*	*Ounces to get 20 grams*
Brewer's yeast	14½	1½
Milk, dried skimmed	10	2
Peanuts	8	2½
Wheatgerm	7	3
Peanut butter	7	3
Hard cheese	7	3
Chicken, kippers, haddock, beef, veal, lamb, pork	6½	3½
Almonds	5½	3¾
Cashew nuts	5	4
Tuna fish	5	4
Cottage cheese	4½	4½
Brazil nuts	4	5
White fish	4	5
Eggs	3½	3 eggs
Walnuts	3½	6
Hazel nuts	2½	8
Wholemeal bread	2¾	8
White bread	2¼	8½
Pulses, cooked	1¾	10
Dried apricots	1½	13
Milk, yoghurt	1	20
Brussels sprouts, cauliflower, peas, potatoes, spinach, sweetcorn, watercress	1	20

But this is only true of people who eat some animal products – such as cheese, milk or eggs. For there is one essential food element which is almost exclusive to foods from animal sources – vitamin B12. It is absolutely vital to us for making red blood cells normally. On the other hand, we need only tiny amounts of it. A chemist I know used to demonstrate this point at lectures: he would take from his pocket a modest sized bottle of vitamin B12 tablets and point out that this contained the whole of the British population's vitamin B12 requirement for a day.

Vegans, or vegetarians who just don't like dairy foods, can slowly run out of vitamin B12. But most of them are well aware of this possible shortage, and use one of the very rare vegetable sources: soya beans, comfrey and royal jelly. All of them contain minute amounts of B12 – and capsules derived from non-meat sources are also available.

There are several different reasons why people are vegetarian, not all of them to do with health theories. Although vegetarians tend to be more knowledgeable about food values than other people, being a vegetarian is by no means always the same thing as being health food-minded – or vice versa. The main non-health reason for being vegetarian is a dislike or disapproval of man killing animals for his own benefit, especially when it isn't necessary for his survival. Some humanitarian vegetarians limit this view to themselves: they just don't want to have these deaths on their own conscience. Others think that everyone should be vegetarian – and their views challenge our whole system of eating and agriculture. For even if animal manures were not necessary for the fertility of the soil, doing without meat implies doing without all dairy produce: milk, butter, cheese, lard, cream etc. It is true that milk and its products are not vital either to man's survival or his health. But huge agricultural and food supply problems would have to be solved if we all went vegan – the name for people who use no animal sources of food.

A second humanitarian reason for not eating meat is growing in appeal, particularly to young people. They feel that the problem of the two-thirds of the world's population who are either short of food or permanently starving is our problem too. And in a world where food resources are limited, eating meat seems to them a wanton waste of those resources. It is undeniable that the amount of land and money needed to rear an eating animal could grow far more than that animal's weight of grain or other food. The modern battery chicken is probably the most efficient converter of its food into flesh – it takes about 12lbs of food to produce a pound of meat (if you allow for bones). Animals like pigs and cows eat 20 and 30lbs of food to produce one pound of meat for us. Sheep are less extravagant only because the land they graze is often unsuitable for crops anyway. But whenever an animal eats one pound of food that is grown for it, that's a piece of land that can't grow one pound of food for a person. So a larger population makes meat less and less sensible. The more pessimistic forecasters believe that within twenty years, we shall all be virtual vegetarians whether we like it or not, and that we really ought to start now.

A third non-health motive for vegetarianism is far more common than most people would think. There are plenty of people who just don't like meat or fish. The taste, the look of it raw, the thought of it . . . they are either not interested or positively repelled. Many small children worry their parents because they won't willingly eat meat. They are usually persuaded to eat it, but there is no evidence whatever that this is a praiseworthy or necessary piece of propaganda.

People are vegetarians for health reasons for one or more of the following reasons:

1. When we digest meat or fish, waste substances are produced which could be irritants to the body if they are not detoxified by the liver. These may be dangerous to us if they are re-absorbed. Some vegetarians argue that man's digestive canal is not suited to meat-eating, because it is so very long. This means that meat and fish stay too long inside us, giving time for them to putrefy and for their waste products to be re-absorbed.
2. Almost all food poisoning is caused by meat or meat products. Eliminating these from our lives cuts out the major source of tummy upsets, trivial and serious. Who knows the long term consequences of such episodes?
3. The cruelty to animals involved in keeping them enclosed in cramped conditions, under artificial lights with synthetic foods, affronts almost anyone, meat-eater or no, who has seen it. Travelling to market and waiting at slaughterhouses can be terrifying experiences for animals – experiences which would horrify us if we thought of our household pets in that situation. Factory farming also provides perhaps the strongest health reason for not

eating meat. The crowded conditions under which animals are kept increase the occurrence of disease. The modern farmer's answer is to give drugs and vaccinations as a preventive as well as a curative measure. A single animal may be dosed dozens of times a year, and residues of such drugs cannot be excluded from the meat as it arrives in the butcher's shop. To these are added the residues of substances given to animals to increase the farmer's productivity. Hormones which make animals put on weight quickly are controlled, but not tightly enough to ensure that the consumer does not eat them too.

4. Eating a lot of protein accelerates development in animals. All well and good, you might think. But unfortunately, this applies not only to the growth of young animals and people, but also to the ageing process. This is in direct contradiction to the common idea that a high level of protein is desirable and helps to maintain youthfulness. As our television advertisements demonstrate, 'high in protein' is still the ultimate praise one can bestow on a food product. It's the central feature of publicity campaigns for bread, cheese, milk, cottage cheese, peanuts. Of course they are all good sources of protein. But man doesn't live by protein alone.

   Although we all need a certain amount of protein, nutritionists are now backpedalling as fast as they can on their theories of how much protein we need. Their current way of thinking is 'look after the calories and the protein will look after itself'. They've realized that in underdeveloped countries, giving people protein when they haven't enough calories is an expensive waste. The body will just convert the proteins into energy, so you might as well have fed them cheaper carbohydrates in the first place. In the West, estimates of how many grams of protein we need a day have been revised downwards. In 1974, the US National Academy of Sciences issued lower recommended allowances for daily protein intake, cutting the level for men from 70gms to 54gms per day, for women from 58 to 46gms, for boys of fifteen to eighteen from 85 to 54gms a day. All these figures still have hefty built-in safety margins. In Britain, the most recent list of recommended daily allowances dates from 1969, and our recommended protein intakes stand at 65 grams for sedentary men to 93 for very active, 55gms for

> most women, 75 for boys of fifteen to eighteen, 58gms for girls the same age. In other words, we don't seem to have caught up with the latest thinking. It all goes to rub in the fact that nobody knows exactly how much protein we need.

But perhaps we don't trust the nutritionists. After all, they are now changing their views . . . they might change them again. There is, however, a more convincing demonstration that a high protein diet is not necessary to mental or physical health. There are certain communities in the world which have become celebrated because so many of their citizens reach extreme old age without losing faculties which we expect to lose decades earlier. The most famous are the Hunzas of North India, the people of Vilcabamba in Ecuador and some communities of Eastern parts of the USSR. In all these countries, people of over ninety are far more common than in the Western world. But more important, in their old age, these people are living physically active, mentally alert, enjoyable lives.

There are many factors which could play a part in this admirable state of health: clean air, high altitude, the minerals in their water, unrefined foods, a lot of exercise and heredity. We can't prove which or which combination is the key. But what these people do prove is that a high protein diet is not one of these favourable factors. Without exception, they eat far less protein than we would think normal. Instead, they eat a lot of cereals, vegetables and beans. They also consume fewer calories a day than we do – and that probably is an important factor in their longevity. It obviously helps their health that they don't get fat – for a start, it gives the body less work to do.

We can't prove that these people's low level of protein helps them live long and well. But it is known that protein speeds up the body's metabolic rate, the rate at which our liver, enzymes and digestive system works. Too much protein may therefore harm us, as well as being expensive and wasteful.

How much is too much? Again, nobody knows exactly, but if we keep our protein down to ten per cent of our total calorie intake, we can be sure we shall be in the right range. On an average British diet of 2,500 calories a day, that means that protein need at the most supply no more than 250 calories. Four calories are supplied by each gram of protein we eat, so that means we need no more than 63 grams of protein a day. The menu below shows how that might be built up – without meat.

Protein in a meatless day

		approximately protein grams
Breakfast	Soaked dried apricots (2oz)	3
	5oz plain yoghurt	5
	1oz wheat germ	7
	Milk in tea or coffee (2oz)	2
		17
	or	
	1 poached egg	7
	2 slices wholemeal toast (2¼oz)	6
	Bran (½oz)	2½
	Milk in tea or coffee (2oz)	2
	1 4oz apple	½
		18
Lunch	Welsh rarebit (with 2oz cheese)	18
	Mixed salad (5oz)	1½
	1oz almonds	5¾
		25¼
Supper	Mushroom casserole (6oz)	11
	Baked potatoes (8oz)	8
	Cauliflower or similar vegetable (4oz)	4
	Yoghurt with fruit (5oz)	5
	Milk in tea or coffee (2oz)	2
		30
Total for day	73¼ or 72¼ according to breakfast	

A vegetarian diet normally contains less fat, which is good because people in the West eat too much of this most calorie-laden of all foods. Vegetarians eat very little animal fat at all (only that in dairy produce – and most vegetarians choose vegetable margarine in perference to butter); and it is animal fat which is linked with heart disease. Measurements have been made of the blood cholesterol of vegetarians: it is much lower than average. The heart attack rates of certain vegetarian religious groups in America and in Europe are also much below average.

However unjust it is, the fact is that to most people in Britain, vegetarians are an oddity. Vegetarians are perpetually coping with the question 'why'. This may sound a simple query, easily answered, but often it isn't. Again completely mistakenly, people who are not vegetarian seem to feel challenged when they meet someone who is. Perhaps they feel that the vegetarian considers their meat-eating immoral, rather than that he merely wishes to abstain. Perhaps they assume that he or she is being positively revolted by each meaty morsel that passes their lips! In any case, they often tend to be both defensive and aggressive. Many a vegetarian's evening out has been dominated by a fierce debate on his eating habits. Some vegetarians, the ones who believe that eating animals is morally and/or ecologically wrong, may welcome this opportunity to publicize their views. Others would just like to get on with their meal in peace! There seems to be only one answer that silences the questioners: 'it's my religion'.

Second to this curious but common resentment which the vegetarian must cope with come the practical problems. Again, the vegetarian is the odd one out. In spite of the sizable number of vegetarians in Britain, they are rarely catered for as a matter of course. This means that the vegetarian must often make special arrangements for vegetarian food to be available if he is eating away from home. Hostesses have to be informed in advance, so must schools, airlines, hospitals, the firm's Christmas party caterers, a package tour hotel . . . Although people are usually helpful, it's another little complication in life. Thinking ahead can be skipped, but the result is likely either to be an unhappy hostess who wished she had known, or a steady diet of cheese salads and omelettes(for egg-eating vegetarians).

Nor does the fact that people want to help mean that they always know how. It is amazing how many people forget that steaks and fish are not the only items that vegetarians won't eat – and forget about meat stock in soup, lard in pastry and even the prawns in the avocado pear. It is the general *attitude* that is at fault, not the person who simply does not want to eat animal produce. But as long as this attitude persists, anyone who wishes to declare himself a vegetarian must be prepared to cope with it.

Action

Stop worrying about getting enough protein. Watch just how much meat, fish, eggs, cheese, and foods based on these you eat: you can cut down to 50-odd grams a day for a woman, 60-odd for a man. Teenagers need more – perhaps up to 70 grams. To reduce the chances of eating drug residues used in factory farming, make any cuts in the meat rather than fish department. If you want to reduce your calorie consumption, cutting fatty meat and hard cheese intake is the quickest way. In doing so, you will also reduce your cholesterol intake.

If you do want to become a vegetarian, declared or not, the Vegetarian Society offers the best information about the practicalities. They have leaflets on what constitutes a balanced week's vegetarian menus, on recipes, on food values. For ethically-motivated vegetarians, their handbook contains a list of which brands of many products, from alcohol to toiletries, are free from animal ingredients. The Society's address is Parkdale, Dunham Road, Altrincham, Cheshire.

6. How You Can Make it Work

Although I've been describing the right way to eat, I know that putting it all into practice does have problems, some of which come from our own habits and inclinations, some from circumstances around us. This chapter is about how to cope with the most common problems met in changing to a more natural way of eating. But the first and essential step towards successful changes in habits is to want the end result enough. You must believe that the prizes are worth the effort. So what do you get out of it?

Keep reminding yourself of these three ultimate benefits: first, and most important, you can expect to feel better and livelier on the day-to-day level. That means fewer days when you feel lacking in enjoyment, and life drags on – more days when you feel so full of well-being that just being alive fills you with a sense of euphoria! Fewer colds, headaches, spots, fewer minor health problems such as chilblains, feeling chilly when it isn't, skin ailments, stuffy noses, indigestion, constipation, 'windiness' . . . whatever your personal weak spots, eating right will help your body resist them and recover from them if they occur. And feeling good has a lot to do with looking good too.

Secondly, you're investing in your health for the future. A body that runs well and smoothly now will go on doing so for longer. That doesn't mean that eating right assures us of living to be a hundred years old. There are other factors which may sabotage our health or long life – heredity, outside pollutants, infections. But eating right plays such an important part, that it will also keep your faculties and abilities working properly for longer than if you didn't bother. What's the use of living longer, if you're in too poor health to enjoy it?

Thirdly, there's another big advantage which I believe is almost as important as the other two. But it is far less easy to describe or put a value on. **Eating naturally has an instinctive appeal to most people, which gives a mental, even spiritual, satisfaction.** Many of us recognize this intangible but very real benefit when we admire speckled brown eggs, when we enjoy home-grown vegetables, freshly baked home-made bread or country cheese. This appeal to our instinct for beauty and nature therefore adds to the quality of life, as well as to our nutrition. Food plays an emotional and symbolic part in our lives, just as much as a physical one. As the Americans recognize, it can be soul food as well as body food. The idea that eating sensibly means sacrificing enjoyment from food is the opposite of the truth. It means a certain effort in changing habits. But if the effort is made, the result is more enjoyment of food, both physically and emotionally.

AN EATING-RIGHT DAY

Rigid plans of meals and recipes have little do do with eating right – because a restrictive diet system is not what I am proposing. We're all different, and have personal likes and dislikes, and eating right is simply a way of life which leads us to choose one rather than another item every time we pick what we're going to eat. So the meals below are not a prescription, just examples of the choices that we're likely to be faced with in everyday life – and which are best nutritionally.

Breakfast

In theory, and in test studies, breakfast is 'a good thing'. It's good in theory because it supplies the body with new nutrients after its longest period without food in the daily cycle. Most of us have 'fasted' for about twelve hours by the time we get to breakfast, and many children who eat supper early may not have eaten for two or three hours longer. Breakfast therefore lifts our energy level ready for a morning's activities.

In practice, too, studies of schoolchildren and workers have both shown that those who do eat breakfast perform better than those who don't. Performance has been measured in physical terms – stamina under exercise, strength of grip, etc. – and in mental terms – agility of thought and quality of decision-making. In a study in a steel factory, for instance, workers who ate breakfast had fewer accidents in the morning than those who didn't. The studies also suggested that the effects of having no breakfast lasted beyond lunchtime: the performance of the no-breakfasters picked up after lunch, but didn't quite catch up with the rest of the group they were in. But many people just don't like eating breakfast. This doesn't mean they are natural abstainers – it is more likely to be a reflection on the rest of their living style. People may not feel like breakfast because they eat a large meal late in the evening – so it isn't a distant memory by breakfast time. They may go to bed late, and so be tired and half-asleep when they get up for work. And if they have to get up in a hurry, organize clothes for the day, get children off to school, it is not surprising that they don't feel like eating. The same people who swear 'they never eat breakfast' may tuck into a hearty morning meal when they are away on holiday – rested and not in a rush, and with someone else making it. And if they can move their evening meal to an earlier time, so that they feel hungry at breakfast and rearrange their morning, this early meal will 'lift' mood and performance.

But there remain some people who never feel like breakfast no matter what. They are often the 'owls' – the people whose daily rhythm would have them up most of the night, and sleeping late each day, were it not for the requirements of our nine-to-five society. If you don't feel like breakfast, you shouldn't force yourself. That's true of all meals.

A good breakfast doesn't need to be a large one. But it does need to be like other meals in providing a balance of nutrients: some carbohydrate, some protein and a little fat, some fibre, some vitamins and minerals. Here are some suggestions. There isn't such a thing as a perfect breakfast for everyone, but you may find there is one for you – one that you enjoy eating, is easy to make, and which you find gives you morning-long energy and good temper.

'Ordinary' breakfasts	**What's wrong?**
⋆ refined cereal, often sugar-coated, with milk and sugar. Sweetened tea or coffee.	⋆ over-processed cereal has no roughage, few vitamins or minerals. Milk is fine, but this breakfast is sugar-laden.
⋆ white toast, spread thickly with butter or margarine and jam or marmalade.	⋆ white bread gives additives, but little roughage; minerals and some vitamins lost. Thick spread of fat pushes up calorie count (fat 220–50 calories per

	ounce), and jam or marmalade are two-thirds sugar, often contain artificial colour and preservative, but little fruit.
★ bacon and eggs, toast, butter and marmalade.	★ unless bacon is grilled and eggs poached, fat in this meal is high. Rest of meal: see comments above.

Recommendations

★ a large boiled or poached egg on wholemeal toast, thinly spread with butter or margarine. An orange or glass of orange juice (about 250 calories).

★ six ounces of low fat, natural yoghurt, with half an ounce of wheat germ, one teaspoon of honey and lots of fresh, chopped fruit (about 250 calories).

★ one ounce of muesli, soaked overnight in water or two ounces each of milk and fruit juice, with a freshly chopped piece of fruit (about 220 calories).

★ one ounce of bran cereal, with four ounces of milk, one ounce of sultanas and a chopped apple, pear or other fruit (about 270 calories).

★ two slices of wholemeal toast (one ounce each), very lightly spread with butter or margarine, with either one ounce of honey or home-made fruit spread, Marmite, one ounce Dutch cheese or three ounces cottage cheese, or two ounces kipper or tuna fish (about 260 calories, except with Marmite, or fruit spread when only 200 calories).

★ porridge made with one ounce of oats and water, served with a little sea salt or a spoonful of honey, molasses or treacle, or home-made fruit spread (about 115 calories with salt, 135 with fruit spread, 197 with other toppings).

In general: a healthy breakfast is low in fat and sugar, but contributes energy, protein, vitamins, minerals and roughage. By sticking to unprocessed foods, you get maximum nutrient value, but minimum additives.

Main meals

More and more people in the West eat their main meal of the day in the evening. It is a natural trend in a society where we wish to maintain the valuable social qualities of meals, and where most of us eat lunch at or near work. From a nutritional point of view, however, it's a regrettable trend. It's illogical to provide our bodies with their largest load of energy shortly before going to bed, and at the time of the day when we are least likely to use the energy up. From an eating-right point of view, we should try to divorce the social benefits of meals from their size, to feed on affection, not on large platefuls. This is often what our tummies tell us to do, particularly if we are tired or tense at the end of the day, but the meal is there, so we eat it.

One way round the problem is to make the evening meal our salad meal of the day. This makes it lighter in calories, but can leave it sizable. However, in many Western households, salad meals are not really considered meals at all: 'rabbit food', 'not satisfying' and 'cold food isn't a proper meal' are some of the criticisms the salad-fan is faced with. Therefore, elevating the status of salads is the way to get them accepted: making them more inventive, more tasy and more attractive-looking.

In my opinion, anyone who wants to eat right has to become a salad-maker of ingenuity and taste. But little skill is involved. If your idea of a salad is a traditional English combination of two limp lettuce leaves, a sliced tomato, a spring onion, a few radishes and a piece of pickled beetroot, you will find it worth investing in a book of salad recipes. There are plenty of books devoted to salad mixtures, and they are a good way of starting off. The first thing they should do is open our eyes to the variety of ingredients that can go into salads. You can make salads every day of the year, and never touch the accepted lettuce, cucumber, tomato, radishes and cress.

Here's a list of some of the options:

Apples
Artichokes, globe and Jerusalem
Asparagus
Beans – green kinds or dried, cooked
Beansprouts – bought or home-grown
Beetroot, raw or cooked
Broccoli
Brussels sprouts
Cabbage
Carrots
Cauliflower
Celery
Chick peas
Dandelion leaves
Kohlrabi
Leeks
Lentils

- Mushrooms
- Mustard and cress
- Onions
- Parsnips
- Peppers
- Potatoes
- Spinach
- Swedes
- Turnips
- Watercress

These are the low-calorie, high vitamin and mineral foods which make the basis of salads. But to make a complete meal from a salad, you can add one or more of the following:

- Barley grains
- Brown rice
- Butter beans
- Cheese – hard or soft
- Eggs
- Fish
- Meat
- Nuts
- Peanuts
- Seeds – pumpkin, sesame or sunflower
- Shellfish
- Soya beans
- Whole grains (wheat, rye, oats, buckwheat, millet)
- Wholemeal spaghetti or macaroni

These add substance, protein, fat, and of course calories. They should be in minor amounts, compared with the vegetables. Salads can also be varied with unusual ingredients such as:

- Bananas
- Bran
- Chestnuts (cooked)
- Dates
- Grapes
- Herbs
- Oranges
- Pears
- Prunes
- Wheat germ

Salad dressings If you want to add polyunsaturated oils to your daily menu, this is the place to use them, where they will not undergo heat which can change their nature. But try to develop a repertoire of salad dressings as varied as your salads. Some at least of these should be low in fat, using plain yoghurt, lemon juice or cottage cheese as the base for the dressing instead of oil. (Try some of the recipes below). For maximum food value, only cut and shred salad ingredients shortly before using them, and dress immediately as a lemon or oil coating will protect the salad from the vitamin-destructive effect of exposure to air. And don't forget that salads can be very different in texture as well as ingredients: shredded fine, shredded coarsely, chopped, cut in strips like thick matches, diced, or left whole and just dipped in dressing before you crunch your way through them.

Unusual Salad Dressings

Apart from the usual mayonnaise and vinegar-and-oil salad dressings (both of which are very high in calories), the following mixtures make appealing salad flavourings.

Yoghurt dressing	Half fill a cup with plain yoghurt. Squeeze in juice from half a lemon, add a teaspoonful of vinegar, a pinch of sea salt and half a teaspoonful of French or German mustard. Variations: flavour with chopped herbs such as chives, parsley, garlic, thyme or marjoram; add chopped green pepper, olives or spring onions; add a large pinch of curry powder.
Tomato dressing	In a liquidizer, blend quarter of a pound of tomatoes with an onion, adding some garlic and black pepper if liked.
Egg dressing	Mash a hard-boiled egg with plain yoghurt or cottage cheese.
Green dressing	Liquidize a cupful of plain yoghurt or half a cup of milk with chopped greens such as spinach, watercress, parsley, spring onions or celery. Season with sea salt and pepper.

Salad evening meals make sense for other reasons too. The aim of a salad meal a day is difficult for many of us to fulfil at lunchtime. English restaurants serving good salads are few and far between. You can pack your own salad lunch, but for many people, it is difficult to find a place to eat it, especially in winter when parks are too cold for sitting out. A third reason applies to families where both husband and wife work. Salad meals are a real liberation for working wives. They are simple and quick to make when you get home, rarely taking more than fifteen minutes to put together. Dressings and cooked ingredients can be prepared in batches so that only the fresh items need to be dealt with after a long working day. Salads don't mind waiting for you if you get home late, either. If you don't like the idea of an all-cold evening meal, then hot soup, baked potatoes or a hot dessert such as baked apples or stewed fruit will warm it up. **Sometimes, people feel they must have a 'proper' cooked**

meal, to show they care about their families. The truth is that a salad-based, not-too-heavy meal shows much more real care: care for your family's well-being.

The conventional main meal is a meat, fish or egg dish, served with cooked vegetables, and a dessert based on sugar and cream, or pie or cake type. There's nothing wrong with the main course here, provided you're eating at least one salad a day, and that vegetables are fresh and lightly cooked; but avoid greasy cooking methods – and the dessert course doesn't pay for its heavy calories in food value.

A healthy main meal is a salad-based meal which is mainly vegetables and fruit, with a small amount of protein or grains. Home-made soup or an appetizer, if liked, can be served to start the meal, and a fruit-based dessert, free from added sugar and low in fat and therefore calories, to follow. (See section on sugar in Chapter 2 for dessert ideas.)

The third meal

For many people today, the third meal of the day is eaten away from home, so this makes it the most difficult meal of the three to arrange healthily: the menu is usually someone else's choice. But difficult doesn't mean impossible. Here are some ways of eating well in spite of circumstances:

Canteen lunches: there's nothing basically wrong with meat-and-two-veg. lunches, if it weren't for the way that many canteens overcook the vegetables, which were probably dried, tinned or frozen in the first place. If they serve a salad, choose that. Avoid dishes made with pastry and refined flour – too much fat, too few vitamins, zero roughage. Avoid sausages for the same reasons. If available, plain meat, fish, eggs or cheese plus salad is the best choice. Desserts are usually hopeless, unless they offer yoghurt. If they do, ask if they'll stock plain yoghurt for your benefit. Cheese, a wholemeal crispbread such as Ryvita and salad may be a possibility. Or you may be able to follow a canteen main course with a piece of fruit, supplied by you if necessary. People may think you're funny or fussy at first. They'll get used to it.

Pub lunches: more and more pubs now serve salads, and in winter, baked potatoes. Ask for your potato with cheese but not butter. For some curious reason, pubs often serve wholemeal bread with fishy sandwiches, but not with others. If you ask often enough, they may oblige by using wholemeal for your sandwiches, but please ask for wholemeal, not brown – you don't want to put them to the trouble for the sake of getting white bread with caramel. The way that pubs make sandwiches, the amount of butter or margarine in a sandwich is unlikely to add substantially to your fat intake. If faced with a salad-less all-white bread pub, fall back on a small bag of peanuts with or without raisins – one of the most nutrition-packed buys you can get anywhere.

And while in pubs, what about alcohol? Or, as a postcard from a Dublin reader once asked me, 'Is Guinness really good for you?' Unfortunately, the yeast and vitamins much-vaunted by beer-drinkers are only present in beer in small supply, relative to the moderately high calorie value of the beer. Spirits have no food value at all except calories. But a small amount of beer (a pint contains about 210 calories) or of wine (a pub glass contains about 75 calories) is not going to do you any harm at all. Eating right includes drinking right, but does not mean being teetotal. Moderation is what it is all about. If you don't want to drink, tomato juice or mineral water is your best choice. Unfortunately, orange and grapefruit juices sold in pubs are sweetened; the mixer drinks are full of sugar and/or additives. A bottle of bitter lemon, for instance, contains sugar, lemons, carbon dioxide, fruit acid, flavouring, preservative, quinine and colour (in order of quantity).

Transport and motorway cafés: as far as I am concerned, these are the bottom of the barrel for finding good meals. But even transport cafés will make you poached eggs, baked beans and tomatoes – nothing wrong with that plateful. And even a motorway café offers plain meat and a salad. For snacks, peanuts, cheese and crispbread, or if desperate, a digestive biscuit, offer the best food value.

Coffee bars: a sandwich with wholemeal bread may be negotiable with a snack bar you use regularly. Cheese and crispbreads, or an omelette or scrambled eggs are other possibilities which they may be prepared to contemplate.

Taking it with you

Often the would-be healthy eater finds that the easiest solution to lunching out is to take his own food with him. This does not have to mean either being anti-social, getting up early to prepare it, or having dull or boring food. Think positive: with a little thought and practice, it means better food, no looking for somewhere to eat, no waiting in queues, and saves you money too. Packed lunches need to be tailored to individual appetites and tastes: obviously, heavy work calls for a more substantial lunch than an office job. But here are some suggestions.

To start with, it's worth buying a lunch box. This widens the kinds of food you can use in packed meals. Pick one that closes really tightly, as you may want to fill it with slightly damp foods like salads. Don't pick too large a box to fit conveniently into whatever bag or briefcase you take to work: if it is too bulky, you'll find yourself resenting it and not using it. Other items to have handy are greaseproof paper or bags, and two small watertight containers for keeping salt and salad dressing in. I use an old prescription bottle for the salt (well washed out and dried in the oven), and a miniature gin bottle, courtesy of British Rail, for the salad dressing. You can keep these in an office drawer, or take them with you each time. Empty margarine cartons of the flatter, oblong shape fit into most lunch boxes, and are useful when you want to pack a salad with something else.

Most packed lunches are quick and easy to make, if indeed they have to be 'made' at all. Portions left over from other meals shouldn't be forgotten for their 'lunch potential'.

⋆ Ploughman's: wholemeal bread, hard or cottage cheese, home pickled onions or pickle. An apple to follow.

⋆ Slimmers' lunch: as many chunks as you want of raw carrot, celery, cucumber, cauliflower sprigs, tomatoes, green pepper, raw swede, lettuce, etc. In a small cottage cheese container, pack the following dip: mix most of a four-ounce carton of cottage cheese with a little milk, to make a smooth consistency, and season with one of the following: finely chopped parsley and chives, a large pinch of curry powder, a spoonful of additive-free tomato sauce or pickle, a little chopped ginger, or a teaspoon of mustard. Fruit or plain yoghurt to follow.

⋆ Sandwiches: make with wholemeal bread, and either reduce or leave out butter or margarine on bread. Choose a moistening filling, such as Marmite and cucumber; grated cheese, lettuce and chutney/pickle; cottage cheese and cress; cress and hardboiled egg mashed with plain yoghurt; shredded lettuce and tuna fish mashed with plain yoghurt and lemon juice; watercress; or just masses of lettuce, tomato and cucumber. Made this way, sandwiches give you extra vitamins, minerals, protein and roughage, but less fat (because of less or no butter on bread). Choose basic fillings to be free of additives which are widely used in pastes, delicatessen meats, etc. You can change the bread for variety to wholemeal rolls, pumpernickel or crispbread.

★ Salads: there are thousands of different combination salads that can be made, but a few points are worth remembering when choosing lunchbox salads. First, don't make them wet: they're more likely to leak and messier to eat. If you use French dressing, add only a tiny amount, or keep separate until lunchtime. A thicker dressing of plain yoghurt with lemon juice binds ingredients together more effectively. Second, some ingredients, such as watercress, lettuce and mustard and cress, should never be dressed in advance. They'll go limp and slimy. But most root vegetable salad ingredients benefit from a very light coating of oil: it stops them going dry and floppy. Third, for all-in-one lunches, include some substantial, proteinous element in the salad, such as grated cheese, peanuts, shelled nuts, fish, eggs or seeds (sesame, sunflower and pumpkin seeds are all high in protein as well as in unsaturated oils).

★ Fruit and nut case: a handful of shelled nuts, a handful of raisins, some fresh fruit and yoghurt to follow. If you prefer, chop the fruit in advance, add a spoonful of wheat germ, mix all together, and just before eating, pour over a carton of plain yoghurt. The wheat germ adds protein, vitamins, and also sweetness.

Snacks

Everyone knows that when you're hungry, it is more tempting to eat whatever is at hand, especially if there's little choice available. So to avoid the doubtful pleasures of British Rail catering, motorway cafés or ice cream vans, keep good-for-you snacks at hand. It may sound silly to carry around emergency rations such as apples, mini-packets of nuts and raisins, or home-made biscuits, but it's no more peculiar than carrying around a book to read when there's an opportunity, and much less strange than keeping packets of cigarettes in your pocket.

All the above suggestions apply equally to children's meals. Some schools provide such good lunches – with properly cooked vegetables, salads and fresh fruit – that there's no reason to avoid them. But don't be nervous about 'making your child different' by providing packed lunches if school meals are awful: remember that what a child eats forms its health and tastes for life. **You are responsible for forming the tastes which will help your child keep its**

sound teeth, a slim figure, and a good skin, and in later life, to avoid serious and unpleasant diseases. Even more important is that your child avoids school tuckshops – surely one of the greatest scandals of our time. That schools should make money out of encouraging children to buy sweets which will do them nothing but harm seems almost incredible – but it's a fact at thousands of British schools.

The emergency rations I mention above really do matter here. Some children understand very quickly that some foods are bad for them, and others good. If you can explain this and provide alternatives, children will find it much easier to keep away from sweets. If there is a school tuckshop, try asking if they can stock yoghurts, apples, peanuts and raisins as well as sweets. And if your child desperately wants to join his friends who use sweet and tuckshops, remember that potato crisps, while hardly an ideal food, are much better for a child than sweets, because they do not contain sugar, and are more satisfying while slightly lower in calories (about 130 calories a small packet, compared with at least 150 and up to 400 for chocolate or confectionery bars such as Mars).

I have little sympathy with mothers who believe they are 'depriving' their children if they don't give them sweets. Up to school age, a child wouldn't know what sweets *were* if his mother or other relatives didn't eat them or give them to him. It is mothers who are mainly responsible for the thousands of adults who go through life craving sweets at times of crisis as a passport back to the sheltered, secure atmosphere of their childhoods, where sweets were prizes for good behaviour, and symbols of love. Why couldn't they feel that way about another, less unhealthy food? Make it bananas, nuts, home-made biscuits, . . . any favourite food, but *not* sweets.

But I have every sympathy with the mother who sees a child becoming fond of sweets once he or she goes to school, or to parties, or receives gifts from other people. It is impossible to stop children from ever eating sweets. But home is the greatest shaper of habits, and a child who's never been used to sweets and doesn't remember them as rewards is more likely to stay fond of savoury foods instead.

Which brings me to one of the most important parts of eating right: not being a fanatic. **You're not engaged upon a moral crusade, just upon forming general eating habits which will make you feel and look your best.** It doesn't matter if a child eats sweets sometimes, it doesn't matter if an adult occasionally eats 'junk' food, either because of circumstances or because of a long-established love of chocolate eclairs! People are far too inclined to see eating healthily like taking the pledge – an almost religious resolve, to break which is sinful. It isn't like that at all. The more healthy choices of food you make, the better, but an unhealthy one now and then doesn't write off all the good you're doing yourself. It may make you feel a bit guilty . . . but it shouldn't.

In fact, a return to eating 'ordinary' food, when travelling or staying with other people, is how many people prove to themselves once and for all how much better they feel on wholefoods. They may have been yearning for a sticky Bath bun – but once they've had a few days of Britain's regular fat-sugar-stodge laden food, they can't wait to get back to food with more taste and freshness.

Eating out

Dinner with friends or at a restaurant is a growing form of entertainment in Britain. Naturally, these are meals where people don't want to feel restricted by thoughts of 'I mustn't eat that'. And there are times when we're offered more elaborately cooked and larger meals than we'd eat regularly. But the idea of 'eating right' doesn't have to be shelved, because it isn't a diet – just a set of eating habits, which become part of everyday life. When you're eating out, you simply choose the foods which fit in best with eating right.

Eating out with friends poses more problems than eating at a restaurant, because there's no menu. So if you don't want to eat sweet puddings, and know your host or hostess is bound to offer a favourite creation, it's fairer to warn them in advance of your taste. You don't have to make a song and dance of it, just to say, when accepting the invitation, that you feel you ought to tell them in advance that you don't eat sweet things. If you don't want to do that, plead fullness when you reach the dessert course. And if they insist . . . well, either insist back again, or take a small portion and eat it. As always, the other foods you want to avoid are those high in fat, such as pastry, fried foods, anything buttered, creamy sauces and pâtés. That doesn't mean you can never touch them, but be aware, and eat sparing amounts of those items. Being sociable and relaxed doesn't mean you have to eat large amounts of things.

In restaurants, it's always possible to eat a perfectly healthy meal if you want to. Simply stick to the unprocessed, less rich items. Salads, melon, avocado, seafood, thin soups or juices make good starters, with unfried meat, fish or egg dishes to follow. Watch other people's plates for a guide to how well the restaurant deals with vegetables: if they look soggy or wooden from freezing, order a side salad instead. Baked potatoes or new potatoes are better than fried, puréed or chipped. And potatoes are a better choice than white rice or white noodles. For dessert, fresh fruit salad isn't always what it says, but if it really is fresh, it's often the best choice. Custard, made with eggs, not powder, or cheese and biscuits are other alternatives almost always available. At restaurant dinner parties, people tend to encourage each other to eat dessert, when no one is really hungry. It may only need one person to say 'I'll just have coffee', and everyone will be relieved to fall in with him.

Drinks

Coffee, tea and chocolate all contain ingredients which mildly stimulate the heart and digestive system. Coffee contains the most of these, and if people drink a lot of *real* coffee, they are likely to notice one or more of the following symptoms: acid stomach, more frequent visits to the lavatory, feeling more alert or more sensitive to things around them, sleeplessness, faster heart beat, nerviness.

So should people avoid coffee altogether? In my view, this is another case where compromise is justified. Many people drink so much coffee that their systems come to depend on it for stimulation. They feel wooden-headed until they give themselves a 'lift' with coffee – and every stimulant leaves a 'down' feeling behind it. But I have yet to see the evidence that an occasional cup of coffee harms. Instant coffee contains only about one seventh of the caffeine – the stimulant agent – of real coffee. But it can still produce the acid digestive symptoms, which are not dependent on caffeine. Decaffeinated coffee contains almost no stimulant, but again can irritate some people's digestion. Anyone who drinks coffee to the point where they can feel its effects is drinking too much. Two cups of real coffee, for instance, would be enough for most people. As with alcohol, the less you've eaten, the more you'll feel the effects of drinking coffee, and the more likely it is to cause indigestion. So stick to an occasional cup of real coffee, don't keep a percolator or jug ever at the ready.

Some people are extraordinarily sensitive to coffee, and for them, it can produce severe allergic reactions such as migraine and rashes. Obviously, they should stop drinking it altogether. And for anyone who has unexplained allergic reactions, coffee is one of the drinks to suspect.

Tea contains some caffeine too, as well as tannin, which also stimulates. In contrast to coffee, tea tends to have a constipating effect. But it too can be a minor addiction. So once again, don't drink cups and cups of it. The stimulant power of tea will vary both with the blend, and with how strong you make your tea. You can buy low tannin tea in health food shops, and you can also cut down on tannin by adopting lemon tea, which is drunk much weaker. A more drastic way of cutting down on tea's stimulant powers involves breaking all the rules of tea-making, but never mind! Scald the tea leaves with boiling water, leave for thirty seconds, then pour off the water, and remake the tea with more boiling water. A lot of the stimulant will be in the thrown-away water.

Chocolate is not a drink most of us think of as stimulant, but it is. It is ironic therefore that it is mainly drunk as a soothing bedtime potion . . . From an eating-right point of view, chocolate is the worst of the three, because it is only drinkable with sugar, since the cocoa bean is naturally bitter. This and the milk used make it high in calories too. Chocolate also causes migraines in some people.

If you drink tea, coffee and chocolate, with sugar too, they become much worse, both as stimulants and as 'empty calorie' foods. If you drink five cups of one of these a day (one with each meal, with two between-meal drinks), and you take two teaspoons of sugar with each cup, you're taking about two ounces of sugar a day in this way. That's 225 empty calories: over 10 per cent of most people's total daily calorie intake, thrown away on a non-food.

Soft drinks are really sweets in liquid form: sugary water with added flavours and colours. They're just as useless nutritionally as sweets, just as likely to rot your teeth, and almost as fattening. So what can you drink instead? Try fruit juice (unsweetened), mineral water, soda water, home made lemonade with honey, not sugar, vegetable juices (tomato, V8 or home-made), ordinary water, Marmite and similar yeast drinks, herb teas, hot and cold. Soft drinks may be everyday for most people, but they can hardly be described as part of our traditional fare. Doing without them is no hardship.

Alcohol. Where does alcohol fit in to the right way to eat?

Alcohol is a more powerful stimulant and depressant than tea or coffee. The more powerful the drink, the more concentrated its effect. Alcohol provides little but calories. The vaunted goodness of some kinds of stout *is* present, but in such small quantities that you would have to acquire a generous beer belly before you derived much benefit from them.

However, as most people recognize, alcohol does have relaxing, soothing properties. And there seems to be no harm in enjoying these occasionally, and moderately. Because concentrated alcohol is so powerful, spirits and fortified wines are best steered clear of. But wine, beer and cider all dilute their alcoholic content. So you don't have to become teetotal to be healthy – just a very light drinker. And whenever you are counting calories, don't forget the ones you get from alcohol.

One extra reason for being careful about how much alcohol you drink is the additives used to make it. The Real Ale campaign has done a lot to make people more aware of the degree to which alcohol is processed nowadays in much the same way as food. Real ale and home-made beer and wines are more likely to benefit you than other kinds. Hangovers are excellent evidence of damage done to the body: in particular, too much alcohol dehydrates the body, is a severe strain on the liver and lowers your level of B vitamins.

Entertaining your friends

A moment when most would-be healthy eaters waver is when they're deciding what to serve at a meal or party given to friends. They're worried that their friends won't like their style of eating. This anxiety is only natural, particularly when you're starting to use wholemeal flour and brown rice, and may doubt your own skill at preparing them. It's usually a needless anxiety, in my experience. People are very adaptable, and most enjoy new styles of cooking. But if you feel nervous, there are ways in which you can serve wholefood meals without anyone noticing that they are anything out of the ordinary at all.

You can, for instance, serve home-made soup with wholemeal rolls; plainly cooked meat or fish, baked potatoes, lightly cooked vegetables, or a salad; fruit salad and yoghurt, or fruit crumble made with wholemeal flour; or fresh fruit, cheese and biscuits. Nothing in that spread would be strange to anyone.

If you would like to offer dinner guests something more elaborate, there's still no problem. 'Posh' food doesn't have to be sugary, or rich in fats and creams. After all, caviar, asparagus, salmon, strawberries, lobsters and game birds are all irreproachably natural, healthy foods. What you want to keep away from are the pseudo-posh foods: elaborate, creamy, recipes which do their best to disguise what the original ingredients were. Here are two contrasting examples of what I mean:

Posh and healthy	**Not so healthy**
Avocado with prawns	Vol-au-vent (bought cases, filled with creamy flavoured sauce)
Grilled sole with lemon	Veal escalope (breadcrumbed, fried veal cutlet)
Baked potato	Sautéed potatoes
Watercress salad	Peas
Fresh fruit salad	Chocolate mousse
Advantages: no added sugar; three fresh dishes (avocado, salad and dessert); low in fat; reasonable in calories, provided you don't bind the prawns with mayonnaise, pile tartare sauce on the fish, or drown the fruit salad in cream.	Weak points: fat from pastry, cream sauce, fried veal, potatoes and dessert. Nothing uncooked. Sugary dessert.

TIME

One of the reasons people give for using processed foods and generally not bothering with what they eat is that it would take too long to cook from basics. Too long compared with what, I wonder? It's true that it takes longer to make soup from scratch than to open a tin, but it's quicker to make a salad than to cook up a plate of lasagne. **Healthy eating is essentially simple eating, and therefore is often quick.** If you want to make the things you can buy as convenience foods yourself, it will take a long time, but there are plenty of other things which taste nice and are easy and quick to make. As I said about salads, eating healthily can be a liberation from a lot of cooking, particularly from such jobs as making sauces, making complicated desserts and peeling vegetables.

If you do want to make the complicated things from scratch, from natural ingredients, the extra time will be justified both by the superior taste of the final dish, and by its superior value to your body. For whether you think something takes too long depends on what you think its value to you is. Some people think *any* cooking takes too long – and they exist on a completely pre-made diet. People wait at supermarket checkouts with baskets full of pies, ready-made cakes, heat-and-eat tinned meals, pots of ready-prepared mousse. My only comment is that they must be giving everything else in their lives a higher priority than good food (a choice I admit they're perfectly entitled to make).

At the other end of the scale come the many people to whom cooking is a pleasure and even a hobby. They're prepared to spend whole days cooking for a dinner party – and again, that's their choice. The healthy-eating person may belong to either the hate-cooking or love-cooking group – or be in between. If he hates cooking, he'll live on salads, wholemeal bread, cheese, cold meat and fruit – and be all the better for it. If he loves cooking, it may be cheese soufflés, carefully made soups and elegantly arranged salads. But it doesn't have to take a long time. Even making bread can be quick, see Chapter 3.

DO YOU NEED VITAMIN SUPPLEMENTS?

The natural place to obtain the vitamins and minerals we need is in food. But in the last few decades, more and more people have become convinced that the supply of nutrients available to them in their food is inadequate. So they take extra in the form of tablets or capsules. Is their belief correct?

There is no simple answer to this question. Most people agree that if you eat a well-balanced diet – i.e. one which contains a wide variety of foods which between them contribute all the necessary nutrients – you shouldn't need anything extra. This is right, but only if most of that food is unprocessed and carefully cooked, so that the natural supplies of vitamins and minerals have neither been lost nor distorted. But I also believe that many thousands of people in this country do not eat a balanced diet and may be suffering from mild vitamin deficiencies. This notion is pooh-poohed by orthodox nutritionists, who point to the lack of evidence of any such deficiencies, except in a very few cases.

I'm not surprised at the lack of evidence, because I don't

think that slight vitamin or mineral deficiencies are easy to detect. A great many doctors wouldn't recognize them if they saw them – they aren't trained to. And the symptoms they produce – whether it is mouth ulcers, tiredness, digestive troubles, constipation or dry skin – may be too vague to be traced to their cause. **That's why people who change to natural food diets often find it hard to describe the change they notice in themselves: it's too general. They just feel more energetic, free from minor health problems which used to annoy them, and . . . somehow different and better.**

Think of the goods you see in other people's supermarket baskets, and perhaps you won't find the existence of vitamin and mineral deficiencies in modern-day Britain hard to believe. Sugar and fat taking up two-thirds of the calories – but bringing with them very little in the way of vitamins; and processed foods taking over more and more of people's meals are enormous vitamin-displacing trends.

The most likely people to be at risk from lack of vitamins are:

★ elderly people, who absorb vitamins and minerals less efficiently, and also tend to eat less, so have less to absorb in the first place. Frequently older people don't realize that it matters even more vitally to their well-being that they have the necessary vitamins.

★ people on slimming diets. Cutting down on calories automatically reduces your vitamin and mineral intake too. People nowadays eat less than their forefathers anyway, since we need fewer calories for our labour-saved lives. But our bodies go on needing essential nutrients – especially as we tend nowadays to have larger frames.

★ people who eat regularly in canteens, school dining-rooms, hospitals and other institutional catering establishments. They're depending on mass-prepared food, mainly based on convenience foods, mainly pre-cooked and often over-cooked, and kept hot for long periods. Such food is heavily weighted towards refined carbohydrates, and can't be trusted for vitamins or minerals.

★ people who are ill or convalescent, who may have a poor appetite and be given rather bland, supposedly easy-to-digest food.

⋆ anyone taking drugs regularly, including the contraceptive pill. Many drugs change the body's vitamin status. In the case of oral contraceptives, for instance, the levels of vitamins B2, B6, and C and folic acid are substantially reduced, as are zinc levels. Vitamin A levels in the blood rise, but this is thought to be because the drug causes the body to mobilize its vitamin A stores – suggesting a possible deficiency later.

⋆ people whose lives are largely spent travelling so that they constantly eat in low-price restaurants, where the same catering problems exist as in my comments on institutions above.

Anyone who thinks they may be at risk of vitamin deficiency may well be puzzled as to what to take to guard against it. The obvious choice, if vitamins are seen as a kind of 'insurance', is a multi-vitamin and mineral supplement. I would always seek out one where the ingredients are derived from natural sources. I know that most synthetic vitamins are identical chemical structures to the natural versions, but I still doubt whether we've got nature taped as well as we think we have. There are so many cases where synthetic and natural versions of the same thing don't act identically as they are expected to do.

If someone suspects that a particular symptom of ill-health really means a vitamin deficiency, the first step is to get the illness identified. Self-diagnosis is a potentially dangerous game, so go to a doctor, a qualified naturopath who is a member of the British Naturopathic and Osteopathic Association, or a homoeopath who is a Member or Fellow of the 'F.Hom' (Faculty of Homoeopathy) – who will also be a medically qualified doctor.

If your symptom is diagnosed (or not diagnosed), and you are told it is nothing to worry about, but it fails to right itself, it may be worthwhile trying vitamin therapy. Under a naturopath, this can be chosen for you, in a way that most doctors won't do or don't approve of. Never mind – you may be reassured to know that literally thousands of people have written to *Here's Health* to tell us how naturopaths succeeded in curing them where doctors couldn't help. If you don't want to go to a naturopath or can't find one, you must read very carefully about the functions and effects of different vitamins before deciding to take one or another. I have said that nutrition isn't an exact science, but much useful information does exist, and on supplements, you'll find a lot of it

Mineral chart

Mineral	*Amount needed daily* *Best food sources*	*Results of deficiency – and who's at risk*
Calcium	500mg. Milk and other dairy foods, green vegetables	*Deficiency leads to* retarded bone growth, spasms, nervous excitability, kidney failure, congestive heart disease, loss of muscle power. *At risk:* pregnant and breastfeeding women, those taking cortisone and other steroid drugs. *Main cause of deficiency:* is poor absorption, rather than poor supply.
Chromium	Not known	Trace element: little known, but *deficiency leads to* bloodshot eyes, poor vision, poor growth, upsets body's ability to turn food into energy, and is linked with heart trouble. *At risk:* low levels are noted in heart patients. Also diabetics and pregnant women. *Cause of deficiency:* very difficult to absorb more than 3% of amount eaten in food.
Cobalt	Not known	Trace element: few facts known, but proved to be essential in 1948, when shown that 4% of vital vitamin B12 is cobalt. Total amount in body: about 2mg.
Copper	Estimated at 2mg. Many foods	*Deficiency leads to* general weakness, impaired breathing, grey hair, lack of fertility, heart defects, digestive disturbances and anaemia. Also to degeneration of nerve sheath endings. *At risk:* those eating low protein diets, or being fed long term intravenously. *Cause of deficiency:* not known, except that other minerals can interfere with its availability to body.
Fluorine	Not known Drinking water, tea, particularly China	Trace element: function not known in man, though recently proved essential for rat growth. No deficiency symptoms known.
Iodine	150mcgs. Sea food and kelp	Unique in being an essential part of some hormones. *Deficiency leads to* whole action of body slowing down, and enlarged thyroid gland (goitre). *At risk:* people living in low iodine, inland areas where soils are naturally lacking in this mineral, usually limestone areas (e.g. Derbyshire) or mountainous ones (Alps, Himalayas).
Iron	18mg for women and boys; 10mg for men Liver, beef, whole grains, dried apricots, molasses and treacle	*Lack leads to* anaemia, sore mouth, cracked lips, poor memory, constant fatigue, depression, reduced resistance to infection. *At risk:* women of childbearing age, because of menstruation; people with rheumatism and arthritis; in kidney, heart and many infectious diseases. *Main cause of deficiency:* absorption is poor in the absence of enough vitamin C, too little digestive acids in stomach, too much fatty food.
Magnesium	300–400mg. Cereals and vegetables	*Deficiency leads to* mental confusion and delirium, convulsions, mental depression, spasms, and changes in heart beat. Lack accelerates ageing, and is seen in those who have died of heart attack. *At risk:* heavy drinkers, those with high blood pressure, patients after operations, pregnant women. *Cause of deficiency:* poor supply from processed food, stress, eating too much sugar.
Manganese	Not known	Little understood, but essential for activating enzyme systems. *Deficiency leads to*

		Cause of deficiency: not known.
Molybdenum	Not known Not known, apart from water.	Trace element, accepted as necessary for man but poorly understood as yet. More concentrated in hard water, so could be linked with lower heart disease frequency in hard water areas.
Nickel	Not known	Trace element found in liver and pancreas, but role not known. Chemically similar to cobalt.
Phosphorus	0.8–1.4gms. Almost all foods	Present in large amounts in body, mostly in bones like calcium. Also involved in many body functions, including use of B vitamins. Dietary deficiency is unlikely because it is so widespread, but can occur if diet consists mainly of processed and refined foods. Usually found in foods with calcium.
Potassium	None fixed In many foods especially vegetables	With sodium, balances body's water stores, so is *vital* to blood pressure, kidney heatlth. *At risk:* anyone taking diuretic drugs, cortisone and steroid drugs, or regularly taking strong laxatives. *Cause of deficiency:* rarely lack of supply, but often drugs.
Selenium	Not known Not known	Trace element recently realized to be vital to function of vitamin E – but how is not understood. Selenium reduces or prevents the effects of vitamin E deficiency in animals, lack may be linked with muscular dystrophy. *At risk:* new born children, particularly if premature; anyone lacking vitamin E.
Silicon	Not known	Trace element, recently reported to be essential to rats, but not yet accepted as essential to man.
Sodium	None fixed Almost all foods	With potassium controls body's water balance. Excess rather than deficiency is problem in Western diet, and is linked with high blood pressure. Too much very bad for people on steroid drugs.
Strontium	Not known Same foods as calcium	Like calcium and magnesium it is stored in bone. No knowledge of role, if any, but present in everyone's bones.
Sulphur	Not fixed In all proteins	Present in all living matter, but role not fully understood. Deficiency not known. Two known B vitamins, thiamin and biotin, contain sulphur.
Tin	Not known	Trace element, see silicon.
Vanadium	Not known	Trace element, recently reported that *deficiency leads to* impaired growth in rats, poor feather growth in chickens. Very little known, but limited trials suggest that a high blood cholesterol level means a low vanadium level in both diet and tissues.
Zinc	10–15mg. Oysters, nuts	*Deficiency leads to* decrease in growth in young, fatigue, congenital abnormalities in babies, defects in sexual organ development, hair loss and skin blistering and breaking. Wounds will not heal normally. *At risk:* low zinc levels are found in those with high blood pressure, arterial heart disease, women who are pregnant or taking contraceptive pills, heavy drinkers, sufferers from TB, and anaemia. *Cause of deficiency:* inborn in few people; otherwise not understood.

gm = grams
mg = milligrams
mcg = micrograms

in *Let's Get Well*, written by the late American nutritionist, Adelle Davis. Like many Americans, Adelle Davis had an overwhelming belief in the importance of very high protein diet, but apart from that, her advice on supplements is full and hard to beat.

Vitamins and minerals should not be taken in larger doses than recommended on the bottle without supervision from a practitioner. Do not expect the dramatic results that drugs have led us to expect from healing substances: vitamins have much less powerful actions, and thereby get one of their most attractive attributes: they're safe. Sudden results do come sometimes, particularly when using B vitamins; but you should give any vitamin several weeks' trial before you say to yourself that it doesn't work.

SLIMMING WITH NATURAL FOODS

The ideal time for people to change to a natural food diet is when they are trying to lose weight. It's then most of all that they need to step up the quality of their food, to make up for cutting down on the quantity. Natural foods and a natural eating pattern contribute to both aims: they are high in vitamins, minerals and roughage, but low in concentrated fats and sugars.

However, slimming is never easy, or everyone would be slim. And many of the factors that make it difficult are the same emotional and social ones which deter people from turning to a natural food diet. People find emotional comfort in food, especially when it is the favourite food of their childhood. They may turn to food as a pleasure when other pleasures are unavailable – apparently the grocery trade in Northern Ireland is amazed at the freedom with which people are spending money on food in recent years.

The use of food as a sex substitute is far more common than people admit; when people fall in love, they often lose weight because the satisfaction of one appetite seems to depress the other. And there is often strong social pressure to eat. It is worst for people from families where food plays a dominant role in family events: for some mothers, their children's reluctance to eat more seems to be taken as rejection of the family. Business is done over meals, friends meet over meals, parties and coffee mornings – it all puts strong pressure on the would-be abstainer. No diet, however sensible, will work unless the person following it can reconcile the diet with his emotional needs and his daily life style. However, once those emotional pressures are recognized and taken into account, natural foods *can* help.

There are many ways to diet successfully, but they all have certain points in common:

1. The number of calories consumed must be less than the body is using.
2. The diet should include a variety of food, or it won't supply all the different essential nutrients.
3. The foods which supply most food value for calories should be given priority, and the ones which supply least vitamins and minerals the lowest priority.
4. The slimmer shouldn't get constipated: it will make him feel under par, which in turn is bad for morale and may tempt him to give up the diet or use irritating laxatives.

I offer you two ways of slimming with natural foods. Both are based on the belief that a diet should not be a totally imbalanced régime, on which you may successfully lose weight, but which could never become a normal diet. They are simply smaller-portion versions of regular wholefood eating patterns.

Plan 1 is for people who live an un-timetabled life, so that a diet which sets out detailed meal plans isn't practical. They may rarely know exactly where they'll be at mealtimes, still less what food is likely to be available. So this plan provides as much flexibility as possible. Plan 2 is for people who like all their calorie-counting done for them. It doesn't have to be followed to the item, but if substitutions are made, the slimmer must take the trouble to check that the new item is of equal calorie value: it's no use eating a 4 ounce banana (about 80 calories) instead of a 4 ounce apple (about 45 calories). But you could eat an orange, pear or large peach instead.

Plan 1

You can eat as much as you want, when you want, of any of the following, provided they aren't fried or served with butter, margarine or oil.

Globe artichokes
Asparagus
Aubergine
Bamboo shoots
Beans, French, green or runner
Bean sprouts
Broccoli

Cabbage
Carrots
Cauliflower
Celeriac
Celery
Chicory
Courgettes
Cress
Cucumber
Fennel
Grapefruit
Kale
Kohlrabi
Lettuce
Marrow
Melon, except watermelon
Mushrooms
Peppers, green or red
Radish
Salsify
Spinach
Swede
Turnip
Vegetable spaghetti
Watercress

Also 'free' are: yeast extract spreads (but not Bovril), lemons, fresh lemon juice, vinegar, bouillon cubes, herb teas, herbs, tea and coffee taken without milk or sugar.

Each day, choose items from the list below: each represents approximately 100, 200 or 300 calories. Count up to 900, then stop – you mustn't have any more.

100 calories
1oz Cheshire cheese
1¼oz Edam cheese
3oz cottage cheese
1 scrambled egg, with ½ tsp oil for cooking
1 large baked apple, stuffed with ½oz sultanas
porridge made with ½oz rolled oats, served with skim milk and sea salt or 1 tsp honey
1 slice wholemeal bread, lightly spread with butter or margarine
3½oz cooked dried beans or lentils
4oz potato in jacket
5oz plain yoghurt with 1 tsp honey or 3oz chopped fruit
1 enormous boiled/poached egg
4oz sweetcorn
¾oz unprocessed breakfast cereal, with skim milk, no sugar
seafood cocktail (2oz prawns, shrimps, crab, mussels, lobster; dressed with plain yoghurt mixed with tomato purée and lemon juice)
2 4oz apples, pears or oranges
2oz dried apricots (weighed before soaking)
home-made vegetable soup (without fat or thickeners) with small slice bread

200 calories

2-egg omelette cooked with 1 tsp oil
5oz low fat plain yoghurt, with 1 tsp honey and large chopped banana
muesli made with ½oz oats, ½oz wheat germ, ¼oz bran, ½oz sultanas, ¼oz skim milk powder, a chopped or shredded apple
a 6oz baked potato, filled with 2oz cottage cheese
1¼oz almonds or cashew nuts
1½oz hazel nuts
wholemeal sandwich, made with 2oz bread, no butter or margarine, filling of 2oz cottage cheese, chicken or tuna, with salad
8oz white fish, cooked without fat
large helping minestrone or similar soup, with slice wholemeal bread, very thinly buttered
6oz cooked brown rice
6oz baked beans
6oz chicken, not fried
2 scrambled eggs (use only 1 tsp oil for cooking them)
cheese sauce made with ¼oz fat, ½ oz wholemeal flour, ⅓ pint skim milk, ½oz grated cheese – use to make cauliflower gratin or cover other vegetables
6oz cottage cheese
complete-meal muesli: ½oz oats, ½oz wheatgerm, 4oz plain low fat yoghurt, 1 grated apple or 5oz soft fruit

300 calories

large wholemeal sandwich, with double filling of chicken, cottage cheese, Dutch cheese, egg, fish or mashed banana, all with salad if liked
8oz carton cottage cheese, with 1oz slice of wholemeal bread
8oz helping chicken (weighed with bone), not fried
8oz baked beans
6oz baked beans on unbuttered wholemeal toast
Chinese mixed vegetables with chicken or prawns
5oz wholemeal pizza slice
7oz baked or grilled liver or kidney
8oz baked potato with 3oz cottage cheese or 1oz grated Cheshire cheese
10oz baked, grilled or steamed white fish with 4oz baked potato

In addition to your 900 calories from these lists, and as much as you like from the free list, you can have 100 calories from fruit and other foods picked from my calorie list of foods on p.152.

It doesn't matter if you eat your 1100-odd calories a day in three meals or in a series of umpteen nibbles. But if anything, the nibble system is better: it's been shown quite clearly that people eating the same number of calories in nibbles, and eating them in three large meals, put on less weight while nibbling. Don't feel tempted therefore to starve all day, then use up all your calories on an evening blowout. That's the time of day you are least likely to use up the calories. In addition, physical exercise is obviously an ideal activity, since it will use up calories you have eaten, as well as keeping you away from eating more. And contrary to a commonly expressed idea, physical exercise does not enlarge most people's appetites. Indeed, it may do the opposite.

Plan 2

This is only for someone who has an established daily routine. It is repetitive, but that reduces the need to count and plan.

Breakfasts
1 egg, boiled or poached
1 slice wholemeal bread
¼oz butter/margarine (optional)
1 large orange, pear, apple or other fruit but not banana
= 270 calories
or
1oz oats (eat raw or make into porridge)
½oz wheat germ
4oz milk, preferably skim
1 tsp honey or treacle *or* 1 apple
= 270 calories
or
5oz plain low fat yoghurt
1 helping fruit (not banana)
1 slice wholemeal bread
¼oz butter/margarine (optional)
= 270 calories

Main meal 1 = 260 – 300 calories
Large salad made from any green vegetables, carrots, turnips, swedes or other vegetables from Plan 1 'free' list. Use

yoghurt and lemon juice or plain lemon juice as dressing.
Plus 4oz prawns or cottage cheese or chicken
or 2oz hard cheese *or* 8oz plain yoghurt *or* 2 eggs if you didn't have eggs at breakfast

Main meal 2 = about 300 calories
As many green or salad vegetables as you like, steamed or quickly simmered. Each week, have at least one helping of oily fish, white fish and poultry. Fill the other meals with repeats of these, or with shellfish, cottage cheese, eggs or 3oz portions of Cheshire cheese. Once a week, if you crave a particular meat or fish, have that. You can have large (8oz) portions of all these main courses, except oily fish (6oz), cheese (as above) and pork if you choose that (3oz). Grill, poach, bake or casserole meat and fish. Do not add fat.

Snacks and afters
To add to meals or eat in between:
2 pieces of fruit or 1 banana
2 natural yoghurts or 4oz cottage cheese
as much raw celery, raw carrots and other raw salad stuff as you like, without anything added
= about 200 calories

Drinks
2 glasses dry wine a week, if you must
no sugary drinks – no orange or other fruit juice except tomato juice
maximum 4oz milk a day, or 8oz skim milk
= about 100 calories per day

Weekends
If you prefer, you can eat less during the week, and 'hoard' some calories for the weekend.

Non-meat eaters
Because protein is in a less concentrated form in non-meat foods (excluding dairy foods), vegetarians have more difficulty in reaching their protein quota when on a slimming diet. They should make sure they eat plenty of wheat germ, cottage cheese, yoghurt and eggs.

This diet adds up to under 1,200 calories a day – on which men will lose weight rapidly, but women more slowly. If you want to cut down further, choose only cottage cheese, rather than hard; shellfish, poultry or white fish for as many main courses as possible.

The oily fish is important for its vitamins A and D, but on any diet, I would advise taking a multi-vitamin and mineral supplement each day. In addition, it is extremely difficult to build an adequate iron intake for women into a weight-reducing diet. A daily iron supplement is therefore advisable, and to avoid indigestion and constipation from this, a chelated form is preferable, as sold in health food shops.

If you get constipation while dieting, add a teaspoon of bran to morning cereal, yoghurts and salads, to a maximum of four teaspoons per day. But you shouldn't suffer from constipation on this regime, because of the natural roughage of vegetables in it.

Fasting

If you can muster the will-power to start, fasting for a few days will do you no harm and will make a morale-boosting start to a diet. Perseverance is necessary because the first days of a fast usually produce headaches, feelings of unwellness and, of course, hunger. These are not signals to stop, but signals that your body is ridding itself of stored toxins in the body. Fasting need not be complete: most people find fruit juice fasts, which can also include herb teas and vegetable juices, easier and more agreeable. You simply start by picking the day when you will begin, and making sure that you have no social meals arranged for the four days beginning that day. It's vital to success to blot out the idea of 'meal events'. Then you lay in a generous stock of your favourite juices, mineral waters and herb teas, and drink small amounts whenever you feel like it. These will help keep headaches at bay for the first two days, as will a herbal laxative taken the first day.

Believe me, fasting isn't as difficult as it sounds. Tell everyone you're doing it, and you won't be able to back down! Take on a few bets – anything to get you firmly resolved. But once past the first two days, it is very unusual for people to feel hungry while fasting. After four or five days, you can gradually introduce other foods – but be careful as your digestion needs time to get used to eating again. Fruit, yoghurt and milk are the easiest to re-start with. Fasts don't leave you dying to pack away a huge meal. On the contrary, they leave your appetite smaller for some time – so they make sensible eating afterwards easier. Most people find it easier to fast while working, provided their work isn't heavy manual work. When they have time to themselves at home, there are too many free moments to think of food, and too much temptation in the kitchen. After a fast, most people feel energetic, bright and cheerful – just the right mood to continue dieting.

DOES IT COST MORE?

A favourite excuse for not bothering to eat properly is 'I can't afford it'. It's true that wholemeal bread and flour cost more than white, that honey costs far more than jam, and that it costs more to eat fresh fruit as a snack than a biscuit. **But that doesn't mean that eating healthily costs more in total. For the different pattern of shopping means that you save money on many items too.** For almost every 'extra expense' there's a compensating saving:

Paying more	*Saving more*
Wholemeal bread and flour	People usually eat less of it, as it's more filling. Needs less spread or sandwich filling to be enjoyable. Getting more nutrition for your money. And you'll save more if you make it yourself.
Fresh fruit and vegetables	Tinned vegetables are more expensive than seasonal fresh ones – so you'll save provided you stick to what is in season. Fresh are far more nutritious.
Dried fruit	You'll be eating more fruit as dessert, so saving money on puddings, cakes, biscuits, and other dessert items.
Oils and margarines	You'll be spending nothing on lard, dripping and suet, less on butter.
Fruit juices	You'll be spending nothing on soft drinks, fruit squashes or concentrates.

Protein foods like nuts, beans, cheeses, free-range eggs	You'll be eating less, and so spending less on meat and fish.
Honey	You won't be buying sugar or jam, or false teeth.
Yoghurt	Cream
Muesli, or ingredients such as flaked cereals, wheat germ, dried fruit, etc., for making it	You'll be saving on processed breakfast cereals – I advise anybody to make up their own muesli as it works out far cheaper and can be custom-made to suit your tastes.
Sea salt, herbs and yeast extracts for flavourings	No ordinary salt, ketchups, stock cubes or made-up flavouring mixes.
Brown rice	People eat less and need less topping as rice itself has more flavour.
Miscellaneous other fresh foods	You won't be spending anything on made-up meals (expensive, pound for pound), pastries, pies, mixes, sweets, chocolates, chips, crisps, ice cream, sausages, custard powder and all the other processed foods.

I would add to this that it is possible to eat healthily either economically or extravagantly, just as it is with conventional food. You can live healthily on carrots or on asparagus, on home-made wholemeal bread pudding, or on bought wholemeal baked goods. In many British people's eyes, spending more money than is strictly necessary on food is thought to be slightly sinful. I don't share this view: it is, as someone once said, one of the only pleasures in life which can be anticipated with certainty three times a day, every day. If people are happy to spend their money on hobbies, racing, bingo, sport, music and the rest, why not on food? But on the other hand, if you don't want to spend more than strictly needed on food, or can't, that doesn't rule out eating healthily.

To get a true idea of the cost of unprocessed versus made-up foods, try a visit to a Sainsbury's supermarket, which offers the valuable service of a 'price per pound' ticket on many products. It may amaze you to realize that so-called cheap sweet biscuits cost approximately 30p a pound; potato crisps work out at £1 a pound; that tinned custard (milk and sugar and flavouring) costs 23p a pint; and that so-called cheap steamed puddings work out at 42p a pound. Unprocessed foods are not therefore more expensive if they're part of a 'healthy eating' pattern. But if you want to eat wholemeal bread *and* go on buying sweets, why yes, your food bill will work out higher.

It is difficult to adopt a healthy eating pattern without using a health food shop, unless your local supermarket is very unusual. And people are horrified at the prices in health food shops. I'd like to put in a word in their defence, because I know that most health food stores do not make big profits. Ask yourself why, if they do make huge profits, supermarkets don't follow them and sell the things they sell. The reason is because the health food shop sells foods which are not popular enough to sell in very large quantities. If you sell 1,000 of an item, and only make 1p a time, that's £10. If you only sell 100 of something, and make a profit of 3p a time, you've only made £3. Health food stores are in the second situation: they are selling items which are wanted very much by not very many people, and even though they make a little bit more money on each one, their total income is far lower. They also sell a far wider range of items than a supermarket: perhaps 20 different kinds of honey, instead of two. This means storing, and paying in advance for, a lot of stock. That means tying up or borrowing capital – again, an unprofitable practice. But health food stores need to keep a wide stock because that is one of their attractions: you can find all the odd little things that the old fashioned grocer used to have, but which the supermarket doesn't want because their turnover is too small.

That doesn't mean that you have to buy all your healthy food from health food shops. Your greengrocer is the person most likely to benefit by any change in eating habits. But some items – wheat germ, honey which hasn't been heated and blended, wholemeal flour, free range eggs, unprocessed oils, additive-free goods, bran, dried beans, a good choice of nuts and dried fruit (without mineral oil), yeast for bread-making – all these are hard to find elsewhere. If you want to buy vitamin or mineral supplements, the health food shop is the only place to find ones which are derived from natural sources (although they sell others as well, so check the label). You'll just have to grit your teeth, and reflect on the fact that you've never regarded the price of sweets as a con – yet that's selling you something that not only gives you virtually no goodness, but can actually harm you. At least you're getting something worthwhile for your money.

You can also hunt around for cheaper sources of basic foods. A local mill may be able to supply cheaper flour in bulk (don't keep wholemeal flour for more than two or three months, and always store in the coldest driest place you can). Free-range eggs may be on sale at a local farm, or at a Women's Institute market. You may be able to get your muesli ingredients, oats and nuts at a supermarket (but may not save by doing so). Bulk buys of dried beans, grains, rice or honey may save you money too.

In more and more towns, grain stores are springing up. Usually run by idealistic young people, they operate from unglamorous premises which cost them little, and use volunteer or humbly paid staff – and as a result, can offer very attractively low prices on the grains, nuts, dried fruit, etc., which they sell. These are definitely places to save money, but don't imagine that their low prices mean that those of the health food shop are grossly inflated: unlike the health food store, these shops are not offering a wide stock, nor are they usually paying commercial rents or wages. Why should you worry about that? Well there is a reason for not giving all your custom to grain shops if there is also a local health food shop. In the health food shop, you are paying more for some items in order for the owner to continue to offer the wide specialist range he does. In the last few years, specialist grocers have closed by the hundred, and supermarkets have been steadily whittling away at the choice of foods available. Nobody wants to stock those goods that don't sell fast – and many lines just aren't made any more. Do you remember when Heinz used to advertise '57 varieties'? If you want to keep specialist foods available, keep your health food shop going with your custom. Eating healthily can also save you money by encouraging you to rely less on shop-bought goods and to 'do-it-yourself': make your own pâtés, yoghurt, bread, biscuits, and other items that more and more people buy ready-made.

Above all, it pays to remember that an investment in good eating is an investment in health, and in ourselves. If we feel our best, and look our best, we're much more likely to get the most out of our work, and our lives.

Ten Steps to Better Eating

A basic guide to the ways in which you can improve your eating habits and make sure that your diet is as good as it possibly can be.

1. *Watch what you eat for a week and think about it*
Find out just what your diet is like – most people really don't know. Find out how many meals a week you eat out, and if you eat healthier or unhealtheir things than when eating in. Find out if you get hungrier under stress, or lose your appetite. Find out how you feel under the influence of a large meal, compared with a small one. Do you eat a lot with other people? Does your social life 'choose' your food for you? Until you know your own food habits, it is difficult to assess either whether or not you eat a good diet already, or where it might be changed.

2. *Stop buying processed foods*
Processed foods are the main carriers of additives. Stop buying them, and in one fell swoop, you remove from your life hundreds of possibly dangerous substances, some of which may unknown to you also have caused you allergic reactions. Processed foods include mixes – cake, pudding, instant whip, custard, drink; ready-made desserts and mousses; tinned, dehydrated and frozen mixtures; cakes, puddings, sweets. If you find something tinned with no additives – Heinz baked beans, for instance, make an exception if you want. You may build up a short list of exceptions such as tinned fish, unrefined breakfast cereals, jam with no additives, etc. Read labels, and if the ingredients aren't shown, write to the manufacturer. This is a big step, but not as difficult as people think. If you think you're depriving yourself, you'll find it tougher. If you remember that most of the world's people don't have these kinds of foods, and nor did your great grandparents, you'll get more fun than martyrdom out of it.

3. *Reduce the amount of fat you eat to under 3oz a day*
This includes fat from meat, fish, pastry, chocolate and everything else you eat. At least half of what you do eat should be unsaturated fats from vegetable oils, nuts, seeds or soft margarine labelled 'high in polyunsaturates'. Don't try to cut out all fats, because you need some. Get as much of

your oil as possible cold-pressed. If the label doesn't say it is, it isn't. The price will be higher, but it really is more natural, and you don't need much.

4. *Reduce the amount of sugar you eat by as much as you can*
Replace sugar by non-sweet foods where you can. For occasional sweetness, use fruit, honey, molasses.

5. *Eat at least one salad meal a day*
Salads are the least processed foods we have, with all their vitamins, mineral and enzyme content intact. Cold meals are just as nourishing as hot ones, and raw foods can supply food elements we don't get anywhere else.

6. *Change your flour and bread to wholemeal*
With your salad meals, this will improve your roughage intake as well as vitamins and minerals. You should also find your digestive system working more smoothly. For family or habit reasons, you may have to change to wholemeal gradually. If you want to do this, start by using 81 per cent flour (which is only slightly darker) instead of white, then mix 81 per cent with 100 per cent, before moving to 100 per cent.

7. *Buy more vegetables* and use them to have at least one meatless day a week, more if you like. You'll save money (which can be spent on better oils, better flour, better fruit), and you'll also be helping improve the natural food quality of your meals. Don't store vegetables long, don't cook them long.

8. *Make sure what you drink matches what you eat*
Soft drinks have an extraordinarily high sugar content, tea and coffee contain stimulants which also provoke many allergic reactions; fruit drinks have hardly sniffed the fruit, and depend on artificial flavours and colours. Switch to older, more natural drinks such as pure fruit juice, spring water, herb drinks, home-made lemonade. There's nothing wrong with real ale or real wine – in moderation.

9. *Enjoy your new system*
Don't see a new style of eating as a diet, and don't feel either defensive or virtuous about it to others. It's not crankiness: the overwhelming evidence is that diet does make all the difference to how you feel.

10. *Take at least half an hour of exercise a day*
It will help you know when you are hungry and when you aren't.

Appendix 1
Calorie counter for natural foods

Calories per ounce, except where stated

Figures are for plain food, no cooking fat or sugar added, and unpeeled for vegetables and fruit, except where stated. Calorie values are approximate, because there are natural variations between different samples, and calorie measuring techniques are not always completely accurate.

Beans, cooked
- Butter 26
- Haricots 25
- Lentils 27
- Navy in tomato sauce 26

Biscuits and oatcakes
- Chocolate 150–160
- Plain 115–125
- Rich 120–140
- Oatcakes 110

Bran 62
Bread, wholemeal 63
Breakfast cereals
- All-Bran, Kelloggs 69
- Bran, unprocessed 62*
- Flaked cereals, e.g. muesli base 100–110
- Frugrains 97
- Granola-style cereals 130–140
- Grapenuts 100
- Honey Bran cereal 69
- Muesli, average 105
- Oats, rolled uncooked 110
- Porridge, cooked with water and salt 13
- Puffed rice, wheat, etc. 100
- Wheat cereals, e.g. Shredded Wheat, Weetabix 100–106
- Wheat germ, stabilized 105

Cakes
- Rich fruit 100–115
- Madeira 115
- Fatless sponge 90
- Fruit loaf 105

Carob flour 100
Cheese
- Cheshire 90
- Cottage 30
- Cream 130
- Edam 85
- Hard, except above and Stilton 100–120
- Stilton, blue 105

Chutney and pickle 20–40

Cream
- Double and Devon 128
- Single 51
- Soured 60

*In practice, some of these calories are not available to the body, so the calorie value of bran is lower than it appears.

Crispbread, per slice
- Biscottes, average 35
- Primula rye, extra thin 17
- Scanda Brod brown 32
- Scanda Crisp 19
- Ryvita 26
- Ryking, brown 35
- Vita-Wheat 32

Eggs, 1 standard 80

Fats and oils
- Butter, average 225
- Margarine, average 225
- Oils, average 250
- Vegetable fats, e.g. Soyanutta 260

Fish (weighed without bone or shells except for tinned fish)
- Anchovies 50
- Cockles 14
- Cod 23
- Coley 22
- Crab 35
- Eels 90
- Flounder 25
- Haddock 28
- Hake 24
- Halibut 37
- Herring, fresh 37
- Kipper fillet 51
- Lobster 34
- Mackerel, tinned 80
- Mullet 36
- Mussels 25
- Oysters 14
- Pilchards 60
- Plaice 26
- Prawns 30
- Roe 60
- Salmon, fresh 57
- —— canned 39
- Sardines, canned 84
- Scallops 30
- Shrimps 32
- Sole 24
- Trout 38
- Tuna, fresh 37
- —— canned 72
- Whiting 29
- Winkles 27

Flour and grains (Wholemeal flours have the same calories value as the grains from which they are milled)
- Barley 100
- Buckwheat 98
- Maize 101
- Millet 95
- Oats 110
- Rice, brown 102
- Rye 105
- Wheat 94

Fruit, dried
- Apple rings 71
- Apricots 54
- Currants 72
- Dates 74
- Figs 64
- Peaches 61
- Prunes 38
- Raisins 75
- Sultanas 72

Fruit, fresh
- Apples 10
- Apricots 8
- Bananas 22
- Blackberries 8
- Blueberries 8
- Cherries 11
- Currants 8
- Damsons 11
- Elderberries 20
- Gooseberries 5
- Grapefruit 3
- Grapes 16
- Lemons 4
- Loganberries 5
- Mandarin oranges 10
- Melon, Cantaloupe 7
- —— honeydew 6
- —— water 7

Nectarine 13
Orange 10
Passionfruit 4
Peach 9
Pear 9
Persimmon 17
Pineapple 13
Plum 10
Raspberries 7
Rhubarb 2
Tangerines 7

Honey 82–90

Ice cream, natural 56

Juices, unsweetened
Apple 10
Carrot 12
Grape 19
Grapefruit 16
Lemon 12
Orange 14
Pineapple 16
Tomato 6
Vegetable e.g. V8 6

Meat, fresh
Bacon, grilled 120
Beef, average fat and lean 49
Chicken, weighed with bone 30
—— weighed without bone 55
Duck, weighed with bone 48
—— weighed without bone 89
Ham, lean and fat 120
—— lean only 63
Hare, weighed with bone 37
Kidney, lamb's 28
—— ox 34
Lamb and mutton, average fat and lean 80
Liver, average 40
Pheasant, weighed with bone 38
Pork, fat and lean 120
Rabbit, weighed with bone 26
Tongue, beef 85
—— lamb's 52
Turkey, weighed with bone 34
Venison 56

Milk
Dried, skim milk, made up 10
Soya, liquid 10
Whole liquid 19

Mincemeat 77

Nuts, shelled
Almonds 164
Brazil 189
Cashew 178
Chestnuts, fresh 54
Coconut, fresh 98
—— desiccated unsweetened 172
Hazel 108
Peanuts 166
Pecans 145
Pistachio 166
Walnuts 151

Nut butter, peanut 180

Nutmeats
Brazilia Mix, Prewett's (before mixing) 117
Nutbrawn, Granose 37
Meatless steaks, Granose 36
Nuttolene, Granose 87
Protose, Granose 57
Rissol-nut, Granose (before mixing) 129
Sausalatas 36

Pasta, cooked wholemeal 32
Popcorn, cooked, no sugar or butter 32

Salad dressings
- Mayonnaise 202
- Salad cream 108
- Dietade, Appleford 1

Seeds, shelled
- Linseed 170
- Pumpkin 155
- Sesame 160
- Sunflower 170

Sweeteners
- Sugar, all kinds including fruit sugar 112
- Black treacle 75
- Molasses 70

Vegetables, fresh
- Artichoke, globe 4
- —— Jerusalem 5
- Asparagus 5
- Aubergines 4
- Beans, broad 12
- —— green and runner 4
- Bean sprouts 8
- Beetroot 12
- Broccoli 4
- Brussels sprouts 10
- Cabbage 6
- Carrots 6
- Cauliflower 8
- Celery 2
- Cucumber 3
- Dandelion leaves 9
- Garlic, per clove 2
- Greens, average 3
- Leeks 9
- Lettuce 2
- Marrow or courgettes 3
- Mushrooms 2
- Mustard and cress 3
- Onions 6
- Parsley 6
- Parsnips 14
- Peas 18
- Peppers 9
- Potatoes 24
- Radish 4
- Soyabeans, cooked 30
- Spinach 4
- Swedes 4
- Sweetcorn 28
- Tomato 4
- Turnip 4
- Watercress 4

Yoghurt
- Low fat, unflavoured 15
- Fruit-flavoured, average 22
- Whole milk, unflavoured 20

Figures from *The Composition of Foods*, USA Department of Agriculture Handbook, and *Sainsburys Help You Add Variety to Your Diet*.

Appendix 2
Calories Used in Exercise

Approximate calories used in 10 minutes of continuous activity

Body weight	114lbs	134lbs	154lbs
Resting	15	20	25
Badminton	65	75	85
Bicycling (10mph)	60	65	75
Cricket	40	50	55
Dancing, energetic kind	45	50	55
Fishing, casting	20	20	30
Golf	35	40	45
Isometric exercises/yoga	30	35	40
Running – 7.5mph	95	110	125
– sprint	195	210	225
Squash	70	80	90
Swimming (e.g. crawl 55yds/min)	125	125	125
Table tennis	45	50	55
Walking – upstairs, uphill	145	160	175
– downstairs, downhill	50	55	60
– indoors	15	20	25
– on grass	50	55	60
– on ploughed field	60	70	80
Weightlifting – dumbbells	90	100	110

NB For every extra ten pounds you weigh, add seven calories. Subtract the same for every ten pounds less you weigh, except for swimming, when calories used are constant for all weights, because water carries body weight.

Figures from *International Guide To Fitness and Health*, Larson & Michelman, Crown, NY.

Appendix 3
Booklist

These are books which I have found to be exceptionally useful and informative. I am sure there are some others equally good which I haven't come across, but I can thoroughly recommend the following:

GENERAL

The Food and Health of Western Man by Dr J. Lambert Mount. Charles Knight, Tonbridge, Kent, 1975. Hardback.
The Saccharine Disease by T. L. Cleave. John Wright, Bristol, 1974. Paperback.
Manual of Nutrition. Published by Her Majesty's Stationery Offices. Can be ordered from bookshops or HMSO shops, e.g. 49 High Holborn, London, WC2. Paperback.
Dictionary of Nutrition by Sheila Bingham. Barrie and Jenkins, London, 1977. Hardback.

ON MINERALS

Mental and Elemental Nutrients by C. Pfeiffer. Keats Publishing, New Canaan, Conn., USA, 1976. UK agent: Thorsons Publishers, Denington Estate, Wellingborough, Northants. Hardback.

ON VITAMINS AND VITAMIN SUPPLEMENTS

Let's Get Well by Adelle Davis. *NB* My reservation on this book is that Adelle Davis places too high an importance on protein: her recommendations go far beyond accepted required levels. Published in UK by George Allen and Unwin, London, 1974. Paperback.

ON FIBRE

Taking the Rough with the Smooth by Dr Andrew Stanway. Published in paperback by Pan, London, 1976.

ON FOOD ALLERGIES

Not All in the Mind by Dr Richard Mackarness. Published in paperback by Fontana Books, London, 1976.

ON CALORIES IN FOOD

Manual of Nutrition, see above.

Sainsbury's Help You Add Variety to Your Diet. Booklet published by Sainsbury giving carbohydrate, fat, protein and calorie values for all the foods they sell. Available from some large Sainsbury Stores or from their Public Relations Dept, Stamford House, Stamford Street, London, SE1.

ON CHILDREN AND WHOLEFOODS
Having a Baby Easily and *Children's Health and Happiness*, both by Margaret Brady. Faber and Faber, London, 1968 and 1948 respectively. Hardback.

ON NATURE CURE (i.e. the curative role of diet and fasting)
Nature Cure in a Nutshell by Tom Moule. Thorsons, Wellingborough, Northants, 1973. Paperback.

ON NATURAL FOOD COOKERY
Eating Your Way to Health by Ruth Bircher Benner. Faber and Faber, London, 1966. Paperback.
Joan Lay's Book of Salads by Joan Lay. Thorsons, Wellingborough, Northants, 1976. Paperback.
Natural Food Cookbook by Beatrice Trum Hunter. Published in UK by Faber and Faber, London, 1975. Paperback.
The Wholemeal Kitchen edited by Miriam Polunin. Heinemann, London, 1977. Ringback.
Not Just a Load of Old Lentils by Rose Elliot. Published by White Eagle Publishing Trust, Liss, Hants, 1972, in ringback; and in paperback by Fontana, London, 1976.
Rita Greer's Extraordinary Kitchen Notebook by Rita Greer. Recipes for gluten-free, sugar-free diets, all made without processed foods. Published by the author. Spiral bound. Available from bookshops or from Dietmart, Unit 112, Shepherd's Bush Centre, London, W12.

ON ADDITIVES
Why Additives? a series of essays on additives. Devised and edited by the British Nutrition Foundation. *NB* The British Nutrition Foundation is financed by the British food industry, so this book is a defence of additives. But it is also full of information on the uses of additives, and their pros and cons. There are no other such informative books on this subject. Published in paperback, 1976 by Forbes Publications. Available only by post from them at Hartree House, Queensway, London, W2 4SH.

Appendix 4
Useful addresses

For treatment of illness by dietary means, and advice on natural diet. Also advice on finding a local practitioner
British Naturopathic and Osteopathic Association
Frazer House, 6 Netherhall Gardens, London NW3 (01 435 7830)

Clinic using diet to treat illness, with medically qualified personnel
The Nature Cure Clinic
15 Oldbury Place, London W1 (01 935 6213)

Health hydros where you can reform your eating habits with professional guidance
Enton Hall Health Centre
Nr. Godalming, Surrey (042 879 2233)

Tyringham Clinic
Nr. Newport Pagnell, Buckinghamshire (0908 610450)

For advice on vegetarian food
Vegetarian Society
Parkdale, Dunham Road, Altrincham, Cheshire (061 928 0793)

For information on healthy diet without any animal products
Vegan Society
47 Highlands Road, Leatherhead, Surrey

For advice on diet for pregnancy and babies
National Childbirth Trust
9 Queensborough Terrace, London W2 (01 229 9319)

For information about food, food laws and ingredients
Ministry of Agriculture, Fisheries and Food
Whitehall Place, London SW1 2HH (01 839 7711)

Major food manufacturers:

Beechams Foods Ltd
Beecham House, Great West Road, Brentford, Middlesex

Birds Eye Foods Ltd
Station Avenue, Walton-on-Thames, Surrey KT12 1NT

Bovril Ltd
PO Box 18, Wellington Road, Burton-on-Trent, Staffordshire

Brooke Bond Oxo Ltd
Witneys Technical Centre, Trojan Way, Purley Way, Croydon CR9 9EH

Burtons Biscuits
Slough, Buckinghamshire SL1 4HN

Cadbury Ltd
Bournville, Birmingham

Cadbury Schweppes Ltd
PO Box 171, Franklin House, Bournville Lane, Birmingham 30

Campbells Soups Ltd
Kings Lynn, Norfolk PE30 4HS

Carnation Foods Co. Ltd
11 High Road, London N2 8AW

Colman Foods
Carrow, Norwich NOR 75A

CPC (UK) Ltd
PO Box 1, Paisley, Renfrewshire

Eden Vale
Express Dairy Foods
Victoria Road, Ruislip, Middlesex

Energen Foods Ltd
Ashford, Kent

Glaxo-Farley Foods
Greenford, Middlesex UB6 0HE

Golden Wonder Ltd
Edinburgh House, Abbey Street, Market Harborough, Leicestershire

Heinz Ltd
Hayes Park, Hayes, Middlesex UB4 8AL

Kellogg Co. (GB) Ltd
Park Road, Stretford, Manchester

Kraft Foods Ltd
St George's House, Bayshill Road, Cheltenham, Gloucestershire

J. Lyons & Co. Ltd
Cadby Hall, Hammersmith, London W14 0PA

Marks and Spencer Ltd
Michael House, Baker Street, London W1A 1DN

Mars Ltd
Dundee Road, Slough, Buckinghamshire

Nabisco Foods Ltd
Bridge Road, Welwyn Garden City, Hertfordshire

Nestle Co. Ltd
St George's House, Croydon, Surrey

Princes Foods Ltd
Richmond House, Wilson Road, Huyton, Liverpool

Quaker Oats Ltd
Bridge Road, Southall, Middlesex

RHM Foods Ltd
10 Victoria Road, London NW10 6NV

Rowntree Mackintosh Ltd
Haxby Road, York YO1 1XY

Ryvita Co. Ltd
Old Wareham Road, Poole, Dorset BH17 7NW

RM Scott (Ipswich) Ltd
11 Tower Street, Ipswich, Suffolk

Smedley HP Foods Ltd
Imperial House, Willes Road, Leamington Spa, Warwickshire

Smiths Food Group
255 Newark Road, Lincoln

Spillers Foods Ltd
4–6 Cannon Street, London EC4

Unigate Foods Ltd
Bythesea Road, Trowbridge, Wiltshire

United Biscuits Ltd
Windy Ridge, Ashby de la Zouch, Leicestershire

Van Den Berghs Ltd
Sussex House, Burgess Hill, West Sussex RH15 9AW

Walls Ice Cream Ltd
The Friary, Acton, London W3 6AD

Weetabix Ltd
Station Road, Burton Latimer, Kettering, Northamptonshire

Whitworths Holdings Ltd
Victoria Mills, Wellingborough, Northamptonshire

Index